Lip Reading

a self-help textbook

by Tony Edens

2021

Contents

Tables

Introduction

Although this book is offered as a self-help textbook it can equally well be used as a class textbook for group meetings or for online meetings.

Each chapter is a lip reading lesson divided into two parts. The first part contains information about some aspect of lip reading and is ideally presented by a teacher. The second part is a series of activities to help you to take in and make use of the new information.

For those using the book for self-help there is sufficient detail so they don't need to search elsewhere.

For those working in a group whether in a classroom or on-line there is a clear distinction between the role of the teacher and the role of the learner so best use can be made of limited classroom or online time and learners can continue to learn between formal lessons.

Although this book is offered as a self-help text-book it can equally well be used as a class textbook for group meetings or for online meetings.

One very important part of developing your skill as a lip reader is to practise regularly. This is difficult if you are working alone. Ideally you need a partner or friend who will work with you. Someone who is willing to take the time to lip speak the class practice phrases while you attempt to lip read. If your partner is also learning to lip read, (they don't need to be hard of hearing), you can take it in turns. One person can lip speak while the other lip reads and you can swap roles every so often.

If you don't have someone to work alongside you all is not lost. There are a number of websites dedicated to learning lip reading such as www.lipreadingpractice.co.uk and www.storiesforlipreading.org.uk. They won't follow the exact sets of words, phrases and sentences given in the lessons. But they will cover most, if not all of the lip shapes.

One very important part of developing your skill as a lip-reader is to practise regularly.

While practising your lip reading always have a mirror to hand so that you can see how your lips move as you speak the various sounds, whether consonants or vowels. And be aware that what you feel as you say them in not necessarily what you see when you lip read them.

Work that you can do alone is included in the activities section of each chapter.

Summary of activities and their purpose

Mirror Work:
to learn lip shapes and
lip movements.

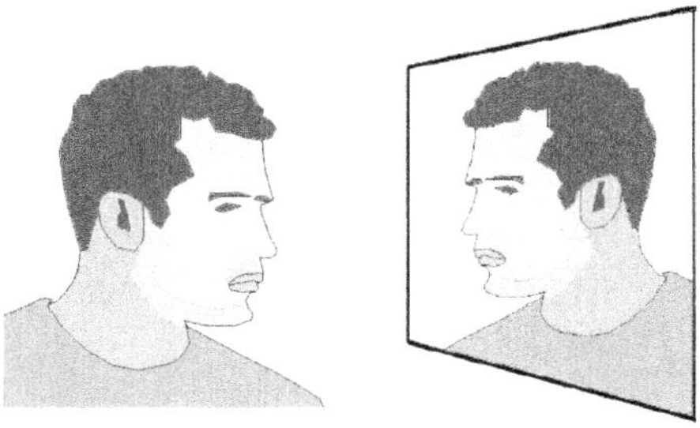

Picture sequences:
to examine lip shapes
and sequences of
speech.

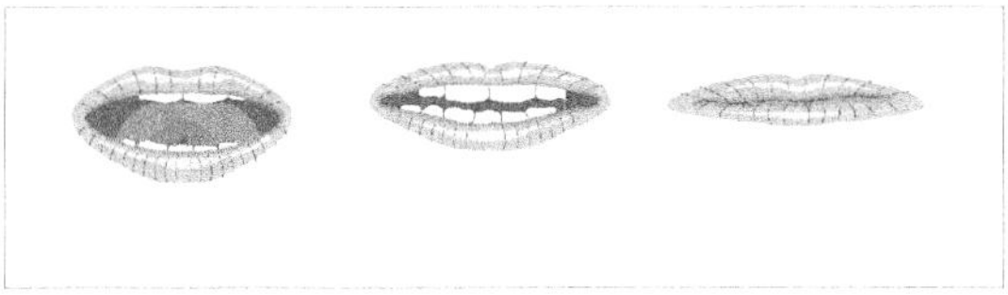

Practising with a partner:
to practise lip reading with
the opportunity for
feedback and repetition.

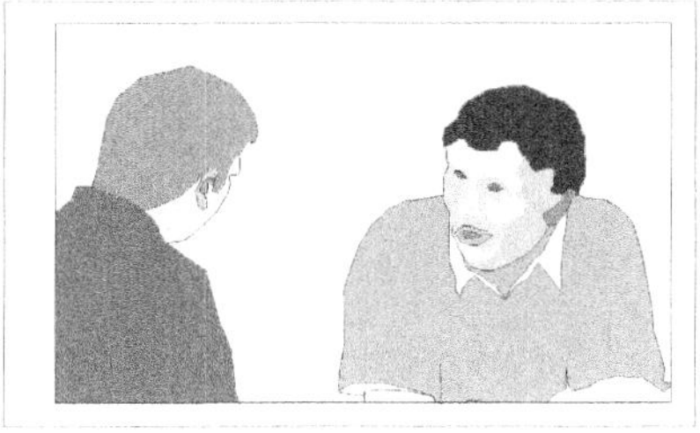

Special texts and puzzles:
to train the mind to
think sounds not spellings
and deal with ambiguity

> *During the* ***WINNER*** *the hedgehog enters hibernation* **SHOOTING** *a place that is* ***TRY*** *and protected ......*

Underlining or highlighting text:
to practise recognizing the
patterns of lip shapes and
sounds of speech.

> ***The owl and the pussycat went to sea in a beautiful pea green boat......***

If you are working in a group:

Whether physically in a classroom or online, your teacher may choose to modify some of the activities by, for instance, lip-speaking the clues to word puzzles instead of interpreting lip-shape text, and in the process, taking the opportunity to demonstrate and discuss some of the finer points of lip reading.

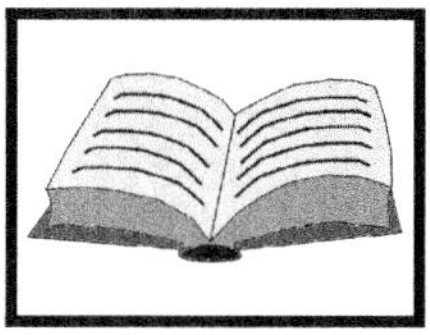

1. What is lip reading?

Lip reading is essentially watching the lips to try to discern what is being said. In practice lip readers use their lip reading skills to supplement what they hear together with any other available information to discern the meaning of the conversation. When we are involved in conversation we make use of a variety clues and not just what we hear. If our hearing is in any way deficient we need to rely more heavily on those extra clues the foremost of which is what we can read on the lips. To emphasize the fact that we use of a variety of visual and audible information, many teachers prefer the term "Speechreading". In this book the term "lip reading" is used to denote the process of reading linguistic information by looking at the mouth and lips alone. It is of course the case that when in conversation we obtain extra information from facial expression and body language as well as taking clues from the situation in which the conversation takes place. But for the rest of this text "lip reading" means reading the lips!

> ***In this book the term "lip reading" is used to denote the process of reading linguistic information by looking at the mouth and lips alone***

One of the first problems would be lip readers encounter when they start learning to lip read is the fact that the way we speak and the way we write are different. Written text follows the rules of spelling and formal grammar. It is accessed by sight and although the message is sequential a certain amount of parallel processing takes place. Spoken text is delivered sequentially. It is based on sounds (not spelling) and has to be interpreted as it is received. There is no going back to have another go if you mishear or don't hear. The words just keep coming and you need to interrupt the speaker if you want them repeated. Lip readers watch the lips and see the words as sounds. This conflicts with what many of us were trained to do at school. Our education from a young age has got our minds thinking of the way words are spelled rather than the way they sound and now that we want to lip read we need to switch back to think in terms of sounds.

For instance when I think of the word "calm" I think of its spelling "C-A-L-M" but when I lip read I have to think of "C-AH-M". That's the way it is spoken where I live. If I'd spelled it that way in school I'd have been told off. Now I have to re-educate myself and maybe find that I'm forgetting how to spell correctly. At least nowadays my computer has got a spelling-checker to remind me when I incorrectly try to spell something the way it sounds.

Spoken language is different from written language

It is important for the student of lip reading to know which lip shapes represent which sounds and your teacher will devote time to dealing with this. The basis of all lip reading is a study of the shape of the lips as they make the sounds that make up speech. So that by watching the ever moving lips we can recognize the patterns that accompany the familiar words, phrases and sentences. The trouble is that there is not a 1 to 1 relationship between lip patterns and words, because many words when spoken, give rise to identical patterns of lip shapes. Note that the term lip shape covers everything that can be seen on and within the lips – including what the teeth and tongue are doing as the words are formed.

The term 'Lip Shape' covers everything that can be seen on and within the lips

The ambiguity problem is at more than one level. It is at the level of the individual lip shape where as an example the sounds "P" and "B" and "M" have exactly the same lip shape where the lips are closed. So when these sounds form part of individual words the ambiguity becomes clear. Words like "pop", "mop" and "bomb" when seen on the lips look almost identical. If you look carefully you may notice that there is a slight difference in how the word "bomb" ends but that slight difference is unlikely to be spotted when followed by other words. In many cases it is possible, from the meaning and the context to decide which one is the correct interpretation.

Coping with ambiguity is part and parcel of the lip reader's skill and with time becomes automatic. In our lip reading classes we analyse some of the misinterpretations that will inevitably arise to show how and why the wrong word was chosen. Quite often your teacher will lip speak sentences that are associated with a particular situation. Things you might hear at the post office or things you might hear at the travel agent perhaps. Knowledge of the circumstance will help you to narrow down what is likely to have been said and give you practice in coming to the right interpretation of what you see and hear. That being said you will still mishear and misinterpret sometimes so you should not be surprised or disappointed when it happens. If you understand why and how the mistake was made you will be in a better position to get it right next time.

Lip reading is ambiguous

Facts about Lip Reading

With Hearing Loss *- particularly when related to advancing years you tend to be able to hear the vowels but not the consonants – you hear people talking but can't work out what they are saying*

Normal Hearing

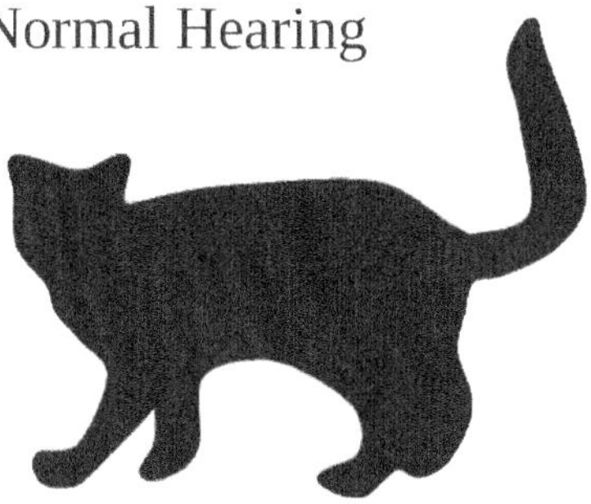

Deficient hearing

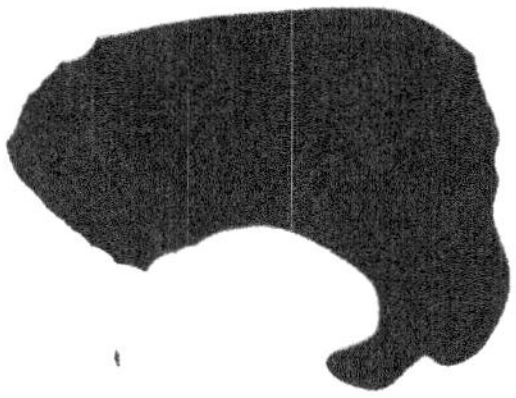

With lip reading *the vowels are usually visible but only some of the consonants – this helps but it does not always give sufficient information.*

Lip-reading alone

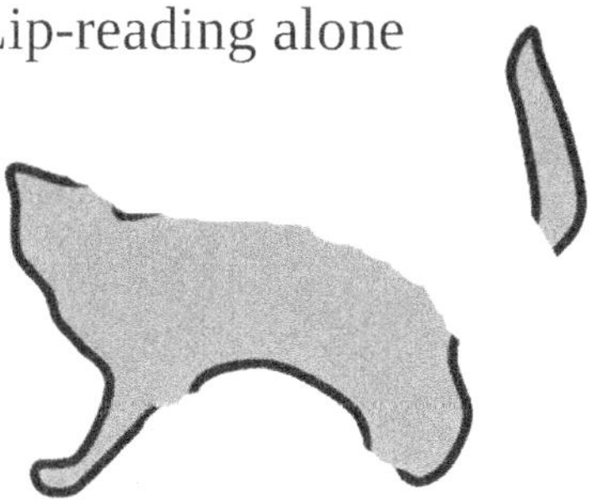

Lip reading plus deficient hearing

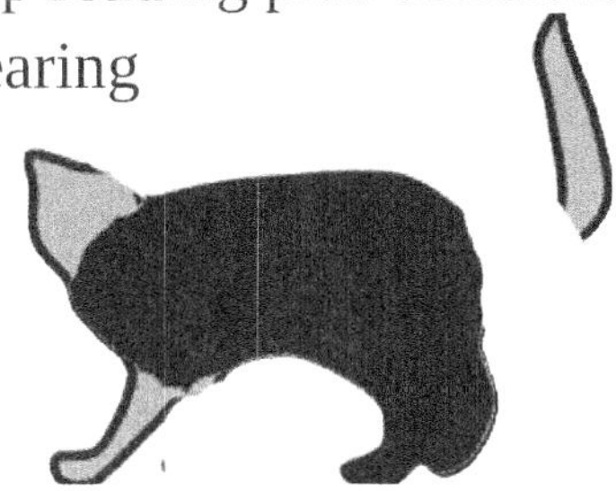

Working out the context *may enable you to guess the rest – you don't always get it right but it's far better than having to rely on your hearing alone.*

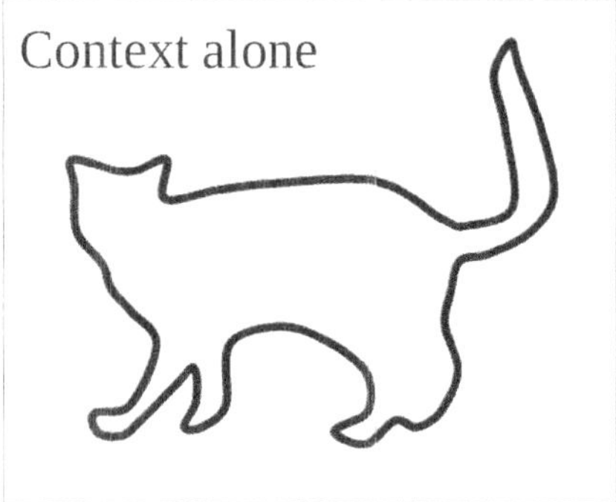
Context alone

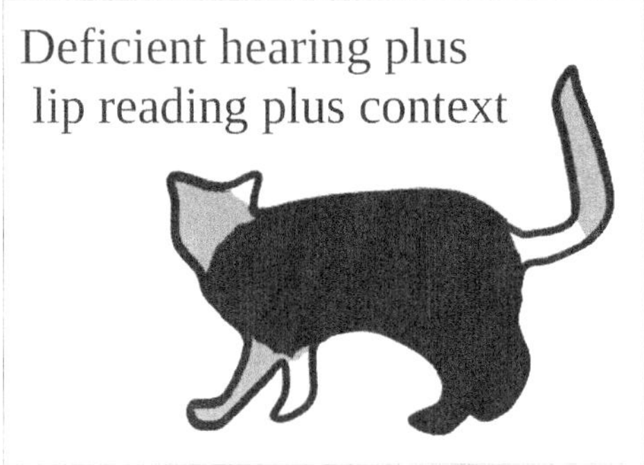
Deficient hearing plus
lip reading plus context

Lip reading works with sounds not letters of the alphabet.

The alphabet has 5 vowels and 21 consonants.

When we lip read we encounter 21 vowel shapes and 12 consonant shapes.

The number of sounds the lip shapes represent is higher.

--------------------------------**Activities:**--------------------------------

Watch your lips in the mirror as you say the following words.

For each word decide:

*Which **SOUND** do the capitalized letter(s) represent?*

(see 'List of Sounds' below);

*Which **LIP-SHAPE** accompanies that sound?*

(see chart on next page);

*Write the **SOUND** under the picture.*

List of Words:

Box	**CH**oice	**D**og	**F**ig	**J**am
List	**M**ake	**N**ail	**P**ost	**R**at
Silver	**SH**ip	**T**iger	**TH**ick	**V**ast
Wax	fo**X**	**Y**ear	colli**S**ion	**Z**oo

List of Sounds

B as in box	**CH** as in choice	**D** as in dog
F as in Fig	**J** as in jam	**L** as in list
M as in make	**N** as in nail	**P** as in Post
R as in Rat	**S** as in Silver	**SH** as in Ship
T as in Tiger	**TH** as in thick	**V** as in vast
W as in wax	**X** as in fox	**Y** as in year
ZH as in collision	**Z** as in zoo	

Pictures of Lip-shapes and their sounds:

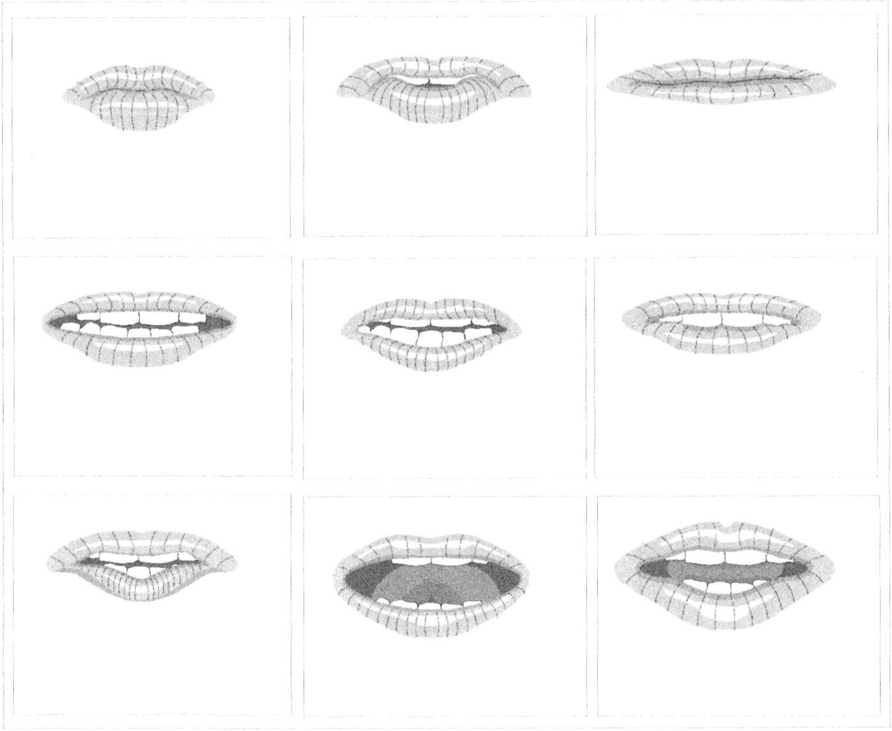

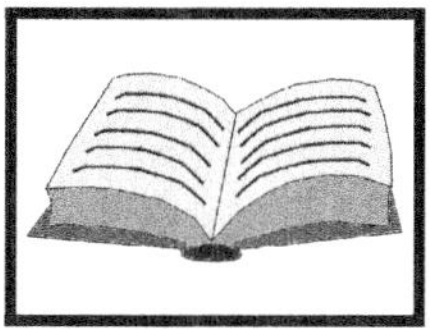

2. Think Sounds – *an introduction to phonetic text*

The patterns of human speech are very complex and the range of sounds the human voice can make is very large. For the purposes of lip reading we identify about 40 sounds that to some extent can be seen by lip readers.

To be able to lip read we must be able to associate the particular lip shapes to their sounds. So we start with the list of sounds and the letters by which we identify them.

A as in Hat	**I** as in lip	**S** as in Silver
AH as in car	**IA** as in idea	**SH** as in Ship
AIR as in care	**II** as in cry	**T** as in Tiger
AW as in claw	**J** as in jam	**TH** as in thick
AY as in hay	**L** as in list	**U** as in cup
B as in box	**M** as in make	**URE** as in pure
C as in cat	**N** as in nail	**UU** as in foot
CH as in choice	**NG** as in Thing	**V** as in vast
D as in dog	**O** as in Hot	**W** as in wax
E as in tent	**OH** as in Crow	**X** as in box
EAR as in clear	**OI** as in Boy	**Y** as in year
EE as in feet	**OO** as in Cool	**Z** as in zoo
ER as in hurt	**OW** as in Cow	**ZH** as in collision
EW as in few	**P** as in Post	
F as in Fig	**Q** as in queen	
H as in hot	**R** as in Rat	

When learning to lip-read it is sometimes useful to be able to write down words as they sound instead of using normal spelling. Writing words in this way will not turn you into a lip reader but it can provide the first step in the right direction. We use it as a means of getting us used to thinking in terms of how words sound instead of how they are spelled.

With some words the spelling stays the same the only difference is that the sounds are separated with full stops (.). So pot becomes p.o.t and pan becomes p.a.n. The reason for the separators is that many of the sounds on the list have more than one letter. “AH”, “OO” and “OW” are examples. So, to avoid confusion, we need to show where one sound ends and the next sound starts. In conventional English spelling the sound of the word and the spelling of the word are different. For example, when using phonetic text: "phone" becomes f.oh.n and "right" becomes r.ii.t.

--------------------------------**Activities:**--------------------------------

Using the table of phonetic symbols above turn the following words written as phonetic text back into normal spelling:

N.ay.m.	K.o.p.ee.
N.e.x.t.	B.i.g.
S.m.aw.l.	T.ii.n.ee.
L.ah.s.t.	L.ah.f.
T.ii.d.ee.	G.ay.t.
H.aw.s.	F.ee.l.d.

The square below contains 17 words in normal spelling. They can run in any direction (left to right, right to left, up or down).

The same words are listed below but are in phonetic form. Can you find all the words?

T.r.ee.	C.oh.d.	L.ii.k.	T.ay.l.er.
M.oh.er.	S.ay.l.er.	S.t.ay.sh.u.n.	R.e.s.l.i.ng.
C.ah.p.e.t.	C.r.i.s.p.	P.o.n.t.oo.n.	H.u.n.t.
F.i.x.t.ure.	T.oo.	T.r.ay.n.	AIR.u.p.l.ay.n.
L.a.b.o.r.a.t.aw.r.ee.			

	A	B	C	D	E	F	G	H	I	J
1	C	E	T	L	I	N	T	R	E	E
2	O	D	S	A	C	G	R	E	A	E
3	W	R	E	R	T	S	U	S	R	R
4	L	T	E	P	A	F	T	A	O	O
5	I	K	E	P	T	I	X	I	L	P
6	C	R	I	S	I	Y	R	T	E	L
7	N	O	P	O	O	N	O	O	N	A
8	T	O	T	N	R	A	T	M	O	W
9	A	L	A	B	O	A	I	N	H	E
10	I	L	O	R	T	R	T	N	U	R

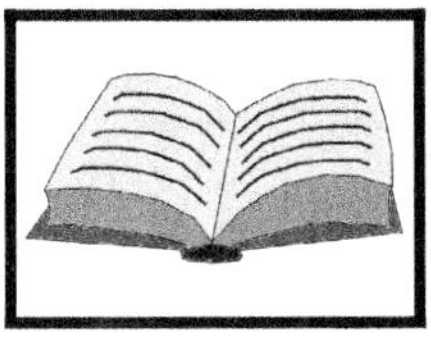

3. Introducing the lip shapes

I have listed 41 sounds that we make when we speak and now I am going to introduce 21 lip shapes that can be seen as we speak. The 41 sounds and the 21 lip shapes is a simplification of what is actually present as we speak. But for the purpose of the lip reader the 41 and 21 will be sufficient. The fact that there more sounds than lip shapes, about twice as many, means that there is quite a bit of doubling up in the use of lip shapes. And we have already noted that the closed lip shape can represent 3 different sounds. Notably P, B and M. (That's Pu, Bu and Mmmmm – not Pee, Bee and Em) Remember we are thinking sounds and not letters of the alphabet. You may also have spotted that the P and B are short sounds and the M is a longer sound. So in theory you should be able to spot the M from its longer duration, but that is not always the case because when our lips are at rest and we are not talking they continue to be the same shape as when we said Mmm. If M comes at the end of the sentence there is no visible indication that the M has stopped.

This may, at first sight, appear to be complicated. But at this stage we don't need to know the fine detail – that will come later. For the moment we just need an overview.

We can all take part in two way conversation and have been able to do so ever since we were toddlers just learning to speak. We may be able to use our language but we don't necessarily understand all the rules of grammar and spelling that make up the formal study of the subject. So it is with lip reading. Many can do it but have never been to a lip reading class. It's one of those natural skills that comes with learning one's language. If you watch a toddler as they learn to speak you may have noticed that they start off by watching the mother's lips and trying to copy the movements and it appears to be the case that they learn to lip read at the same time as they learn to speak, if not before. Once they have some mastery of the lip movements and begin to speak they concentrate their vision more widely than the mother's lips. Other studies have indicated that children born deaf and children born with normal hearing are about as good at lip reading as each other until the early teens. At this stage those with normal hearing do not make further progress with lip reading while those with a hearing problem continue to improve. What all this means is that we are all lip readers to some extent and we are not starting from scratch when we join a lip reading class.

The complete set of lip shapes can be seen in the appendix. It is introduced here to give an overview and you do not need to learn the whole lot in one go. During the course the various shapes will be covered one at a time to build up your familiarity with them. But from the start you will still be able to lip read making use of the partial skill you grew up with. Lip shapes fall into several groups:

The Open group - where the mouth is open for a vowel sound. Examples are:

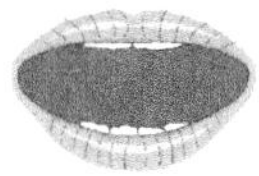

A

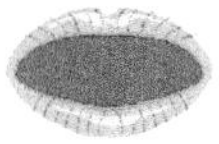

O

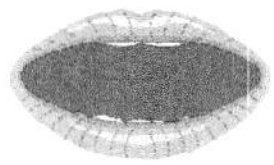

U

The Closed group where the mouth is closed for sounds like M P B F V.TH. Examples are:

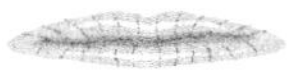

M

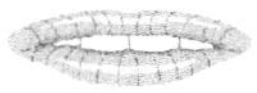

F

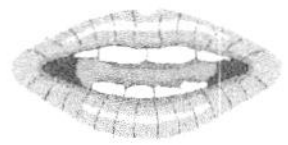

TH

The Cheese group where the teeth are closed. Examples are:

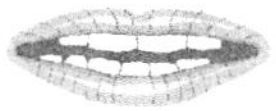

EE

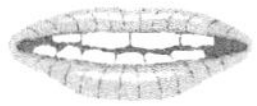

S

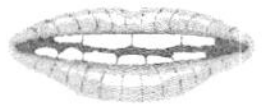

D

The SH group where the lips are pushed forward. Examples are:

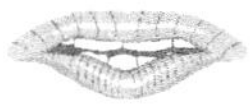

J

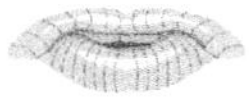

R

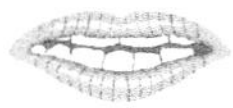

Y

The OO group where the lips are gathered. Examples are:

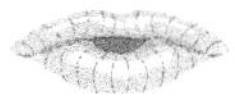

OO

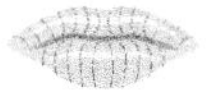

W

Well they don’t all fit neatly into the groups but you get the idea. The images shown here are of course static but when viewed during speech there is constant movement as one lip shape gives way to the next and in the process there is a certain amount of mixing.

-------------------------------**Activities:**--------------------------------

There is a natural progression from the Open group to the OO group as the opening of the mouth changes for the various sounds. In this case they are vowel sounds:
A U O UU OO
Say "Ow" (slowly) in front of the mirror to see the effect.

The closed group are usually separated from each other with vowels.
Say "Mouth" (slowly) in front of the mirror to see how they blend with the open group.

SH group sounds are also usually separated from other sounds by vowels.
Say "woosh" and "shrew" in front of a mirror.

Then there is the progression within the Cheese group from EE to T.
Say "East" in front of a mirror.

The lip-shape pictures show the first lip-shape seen when the name of each word listed below is spoken.

FRIDAY, MONDAY, JANUARY, OCTOBER, SATURDAY, THURSDAY, WEDNESDAY, YEAR.

Using a mirror to watch your own lips as you say the words, can you match the words on the list to the correct lip-shapes?

1____________ 2 ____________ 3 ____________ 4 ____________

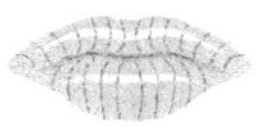
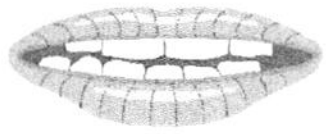
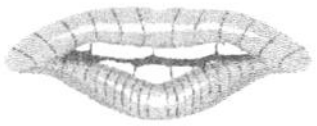
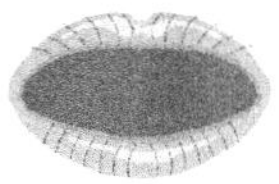

5 ____________ 6 ____________ 7 ____________ 8 ____________

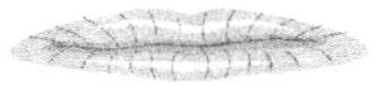
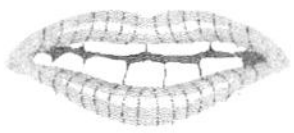
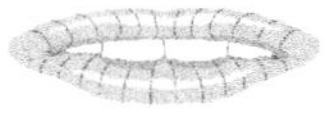
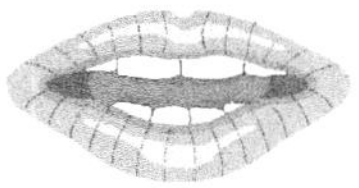

A table containing pictures of all the lip-shapes is in appendix A2. Check the table to see how close your lip-shapes are to those in the table.

All people are different from each other regarding the lip-shapes they use as they speak. Some people have very clear lip-shapes and and are the easiest to lip-read while others hardly move their lips at all when they are speaking. These people are very difficult to lip-read.

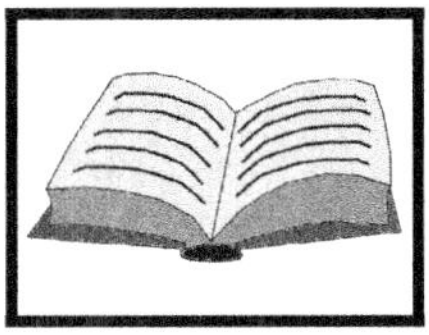

4. Introducing the consonants

J, K, L, M, R, S, T, TH, V, W, Y

When checking the chart of all the lip shapes shown in the appendix you may well have noticed that the vowel shapes on the whole have open shapes while the consonant lip shapes predominantly have visible constrictions. These modify the sound as it leaves the mouth. In most cases teeth or tongue or both can be seen and their relative positions can be used by the lip reader as clues to what sound is being made.

Closed teeth group for S, Z, X, T, D, N

The teeth are visible, the sound is made as air passes between the teeth and is modified by the position of the tongue behind the teeth. Examples are S, Z, X, T D N in words like **S**ite, Si**z**e, Si**x**, **T**in, **D**in and **N**ight:

S Z X

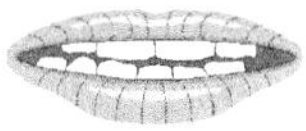

T D N

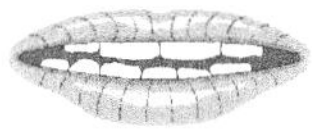

The SZX group and the TDN group are almost impossible to tell apart

Puckered lips group – for J, CH, SH, ZH, Y, R

This is quite like the S group except that the position of the lips and unseen tongue further modifies the sound.
Examples are J, CH, SH, ZH, Y, R as in **J**am, **Y**am and **R**am.:

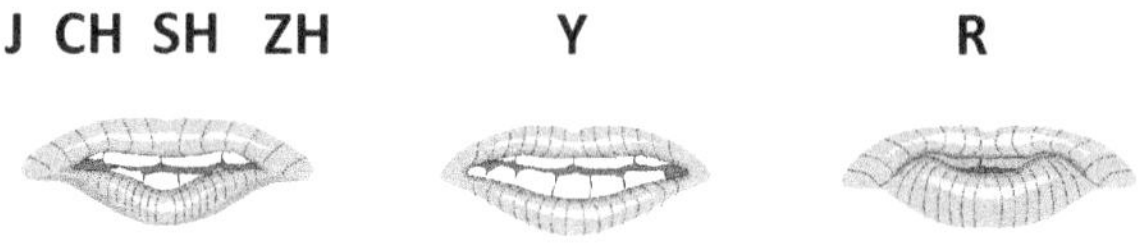
J CH SH ZH
Y
R

Teeth and tongue group – for F, V, TH, L

In this group the teeth and tongue modify the emerging sound at different mouth openings. Examples are F, V, TH, L, as in words like **F**ine, **V**ine, **TH**in, **L**ook:

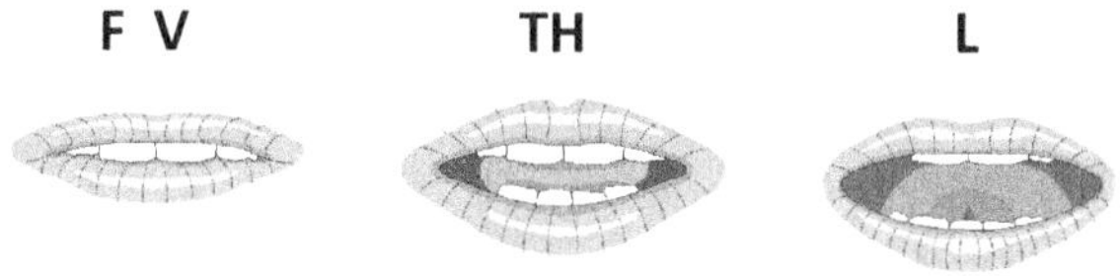
F V
TH
L

Closed Lips group – for M, P, B, W

The lips are closed and the sound emerges from the nose for continuous sounds or released from the mouth as the lips part for punctuated sounds.
Examples are M and W continuous sounds and P, B, W punctuated sounds as in words like **M**et, **P**et **B**et and **W**et:

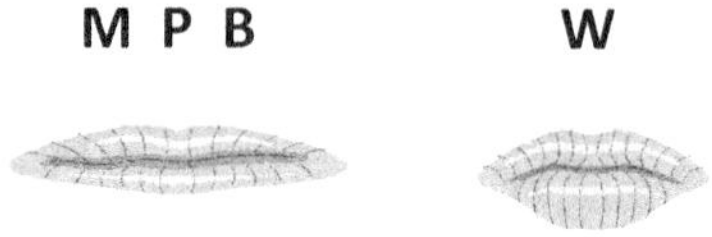
M P B
W

------------------------------Activities:--------------------------------

The lip-shape pictures show the first lip-shape seen when the name of each animal listed below is spoken.

BULLDOG, CHICKEN, DONKEY, FROG, LOVEBIRD, RABBIT, WALRUS, YAK.

Can you match the words on the list to the correct lip-shapes?

1 ____________ 2____________ 3____________ 4____________

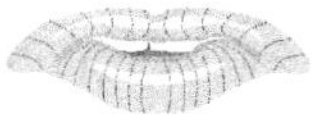
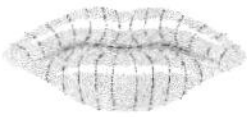
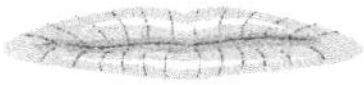
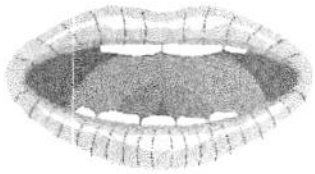

5____________ 6____________ 7____________ 8____________

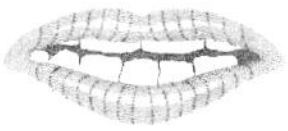
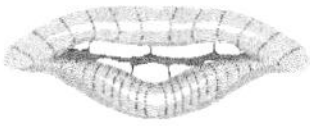
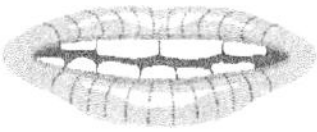
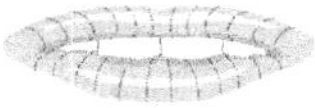

5. Introducing the vowels

A, E, EE, ER, I, O, OO, U, UU

The vowel sounds are made as air is expelled through a relatively open passage. Vowels are liquid sounds and can be held for as long as one has breath.

Vowel lip shapes fall into several groups:

Modified by lips
There is no visible restriction to the emerging sound other than the closing and pursing of the lips. Examples are A, U, O, UU, OO:

	A	U	O	UU	OO

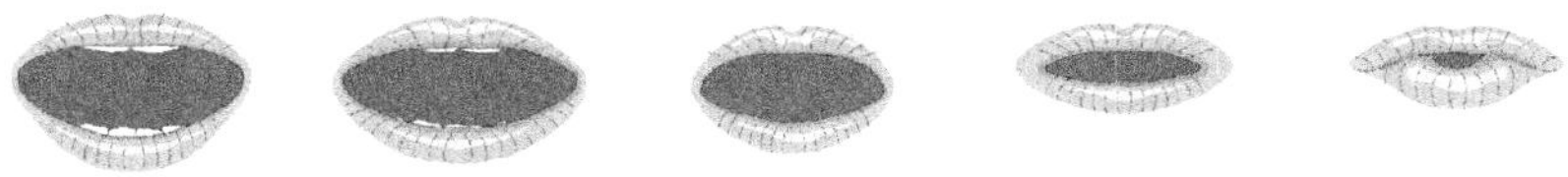

as in:	**pat**	**puddle**	**pot**	**put**	**pool**

Modified by tongue
The lips are in the same position for all the sounds in this group. The only visible difference between the three is the position of the tongue. Examples are E, A, AH:

	E	A	AH

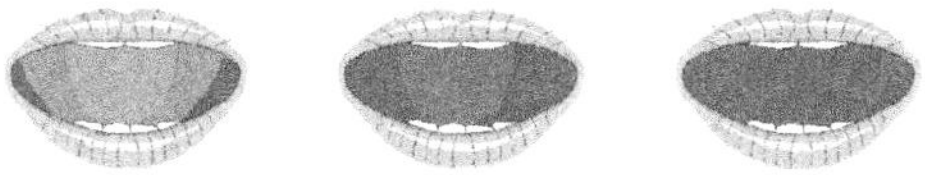

as in:	**net**	**gnat**	**tart**

Modified by teeth

The shape of the lips changes as we progress through the group. The teeth also part. Examples are EE, I, ER:

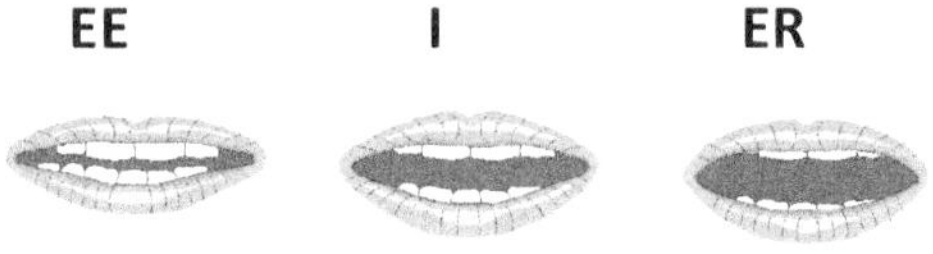
EE
I
ER

as in: **beat** **bit** **bird**

I wouldn't want to suggest that everything is that simple – it never is but the categories are a rough guide that can help us as lip readers to separate out the various shapes and sounds as we interpret.

To some extent the three groups merge into each other as lip tongue and teeth (not to mention other internal structures) come into play to modify the sounds as we speak. But what we are considering are the features the lip reader can see.

The modified by teeth group, as printed above, is a progression in which the teeth have less and less influence and the lips have more and more. So that by the time we get to the ER shape it could quite comfortably fit into the modified by lips group.

With the modified by tongue group the positions of lips and teeth are the same for the three sounds. The position of the tongue is the only thing that changes. For the purposes of this book I reduce this to two shapes that are relatively easy to tell apart, lip shape E and lip shape A. The A and the AH, being more difficult to tell apart are merged together and called lip shape A.

------------------------------**Activities:**------------------------------

The lip-shape pictures show the first lip-shape seen as each of the words listed below is spoken.

APPLE, EASY, EXTRA, INDIA, ORANGE, ORDER, UGLY, URBAN

Using a mirror to watch your own lips as you say the words, can you match the words on the list to the correct lip-shapes? If necessary refer to the table of lip-shapes in appendix A2

1 ____________ 2 ____________ 3 ____________ 4 ____________

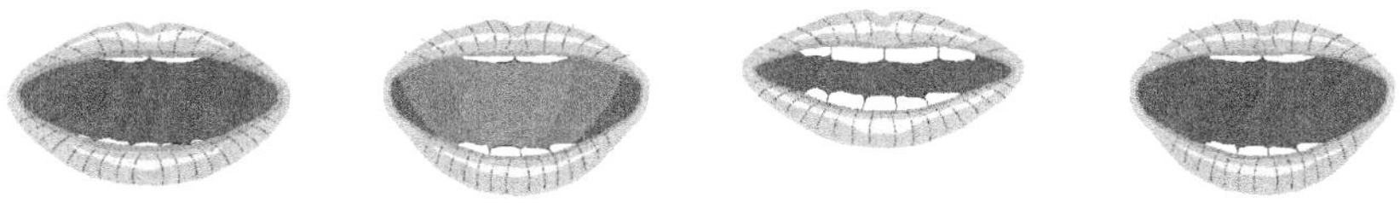

5 ____________ 6 ____________ 7 ____________ 8 ____________

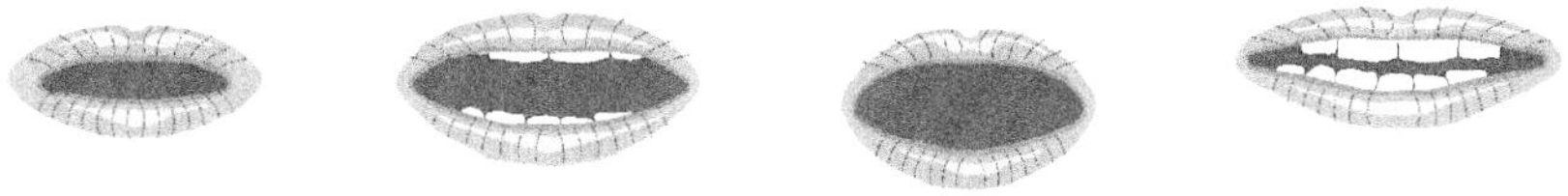

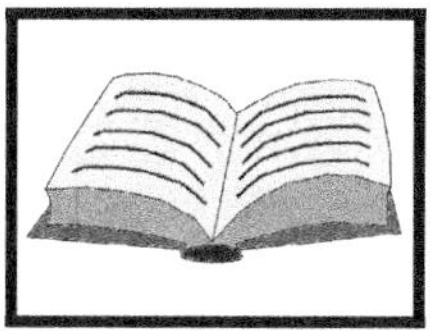

6. Sliding vowels 1

air, ay, ear, ew, ia, ii, oh, oi, ow, ure

All the sounds listed in this group do not sound correctly unless the lips are moving. All are vowels.

For the present we only need to be aware of them and be able to recognize them when heard or when written down.

How the lip reader can see them will be dealt with later.

The complete list of sliding vowels is given below together with examples of each. If you watch your lips in the mirror as you say the example words you may be able to see why they are called sliding vowels.

The name each of the sliding vowels has is given below and this name is used both when used in phonetic text and also when used in basic lip shape text.

AIR

Share	*Stare*	*Where*	*Repair*	*Pair*

AY

Day	*Chain*	*Lane*	*Fray*	*Drain*

EAR

Fear	*Near*	*Beer*	*Rear*	*Hear*

EW

Few	*New*	*Dew*	*Music*	*Hue*

IA

Appeal	*Amiable*	*Brilliant*	*Guardian*	*Associate*

II

Dry	*Pry*	*Fly*	*High*	*Why*

OH

Go	*Snow*	*Flow*	*Know*	*Show*

OI

Toy	*Voice*	*Noise*	*Employ*	*Coin*

OW

Down	*Frown*	*Loud*	*How*	*Shout*

URE

Cure	*Neuron*	*Euro*	*During*	*Sure*

------------------------------Activities:------------------------------

Highlight words containing sliding vowels in this text:

The toy fair will be held this year at the leisure centre on April fifteenth. Exhibitors are asked to set up their stalls between seven and nine in the morning. The public will be admitted at nine o'clock. The fair closes at six pm.

The words below, already used in this lesson, are written the way they *sound.* Can you correctly spell them and complete the word puzzle?

B.ear.	E.m.p.l.oi.	H.ii.	F.l.ii.	SH.ow.t.
CH.ay.n.	SH.air.	SH.oh.w.	C.ure.	F.r.ay.
N.ure.o.n.	V.oi.s.	D.ew.	F.r.ow.n.	R.ear.
W.air.	D.r.ay.n.	G.oh.	R.e.p.air.	H.ear.
D.ure.i.ng.	M.ew.z.i.k.			

	A	B	C	D	E	F	G	H	I	J
1	F	R	A	Y	S	U	M	S	H	D
2	F	L	E	C	I	F	E	R	A	E
3	H	Y	M	P	B	R	O	W	S	W
4	E	A	R	L	E	I	R	N	H	C
5	S	V	Y	O	E	A	T	U	O	H
6	H	O	I	C	R	P	E	N	I	A
7	O	W	C	E	N	E	R	R	G	O
8	E	R	U	R	E	U	R	E	D	U
9	H	E	G	H	D	R	O	A	R	R
10	W	H	I	N	I	A	N	G	N	I

A Sliding Fowl

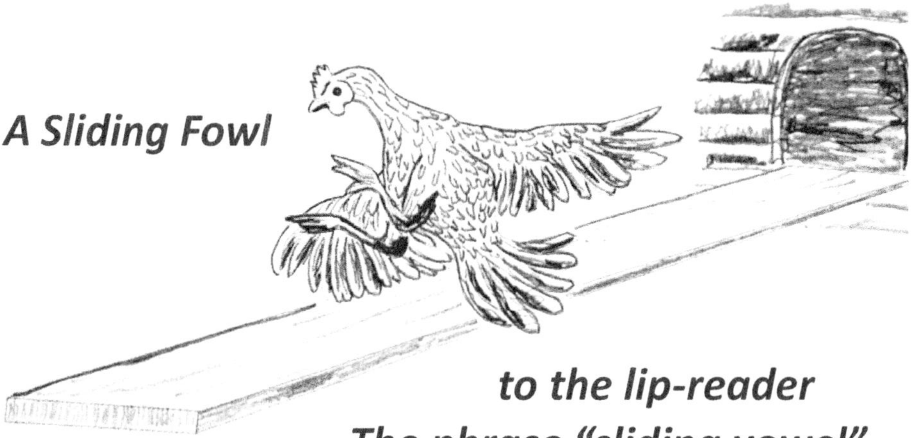

to the lip-reader

The phrase "sliding vowel" looks exactly the same as "sliding fowl".

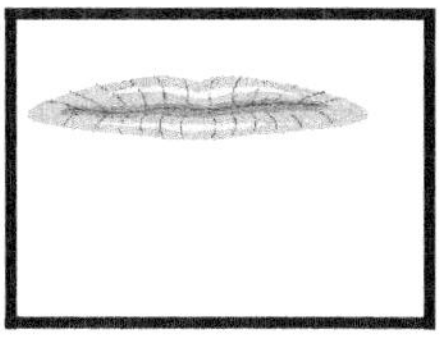

7. Lip Shape M

accompanies B, M and P sounds

The lips are closed for lip shape M just as they are when the lips are at rest. The difference is of course, the presence or lack of movement.

There is no visible difference between the lip shapes for B, P and M though for M the timing is slightly different. P and B sounds happen as the lips part so they are over in an instant. The M sound is made while the lips are held closed and can be held for as long as one has breath.

Watch the lips as these words are spoken:

B, M, or P at start of words:

Mother	Painting	Battle	Moist	Bacon
Posy	Muddle	Parcel	Buckle	Parsley

B, M or P in the middle of words:

Simon	Chapel	Quibble	Fuming	Cabinet
Happen	Cabbage	Rabbit	Tumble	Complain

B, M or P at the end of words:

Lime	Sip	Team	Fib	Drip
Cube	Trap	Leap	Grab	Swim

Words that look similar on the lips:

Watch the lips as these groups of words are spoken – do the words in each group all look the same?:

Most/Post/Boast   Mile/Pile/Bile   Mail/Pail/Bail
Mat/Pat/Bat:

Class practice phrases:

A. Part and parcel
B. Public speaking
C. Mind over matter
D. Broken Promises
E. Pressure of work
F. Pride of place
G. Method in his madness
H. Pass the parcel
I. Peculiar practice
J. Bus pass
K. First past the post
L. Market prices
M. Bread and butter
N. Bright and beautiful

-----------------------------Activities:------------------------------

Match up the words that will look similar on the lips:

Make Pike Beat Meet Praise Bake Memory
Most Peat Bean Pail Boast Bike Post
Mean Patch Braise Mail Badge Peppery
Bail Mike Match

B, M, and P all look the same to lip readers so it's all too easy to misinterpret what is seen.

Modify the interpretations below so that they make sense:

Meauty Marlour
Mread mudding
He wore a clum madge on his lamel.
She filled the mig man with water.
Camming holiday
He went to school my mike.
Please most by letters for me.
Mass the Marcel
Shemherd's mie

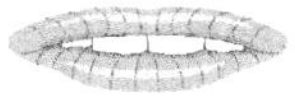

8. Lip Shape V

accompanies F & V sounds

The upper teeth make contact with the lower lip.

With some people it is very easy to see the teeth making contact.

With others the teeth are obscured by the upper lip and are not easy to see.

Watch the lips as these words are spoken:

Unvoiced and difficult to hear:

Fruit	Curfew	Careful	Before	Fewer	Refuse
Refuge	Brief	Stuff	Frequent	Stuffing	Cliff

Voiced and easier to hear:

Travel	Rival	Value	Of	Carvery	Pavilion
Village	Pave	Cover	Over	Trivial	Violent

Spelled with gh or ph:

Laugh   Tough   Ephemeral   Photograph

Words that look the same:

Fat/Vat   Fail/Veil   Off/Of

Class practice phrases:

A. Fast and furious
B. Few and far between
C. Work of fiction
D. Self service checkout
E. Photo finish
F. That's enough

G. Fact and fiction
H. Halfway through
I. Frequent service
J. Flight of fancy
K. A laugh a minute
L. Rough justice

--------------------------------**Activities:**----------------------------------

The words *cover, tough, village and brief* have been encoded as a series of lip shapes – by watching your own lips in a mirror or by reference to the lip shape table in Appendix A2 can you work out which is which?

A

B

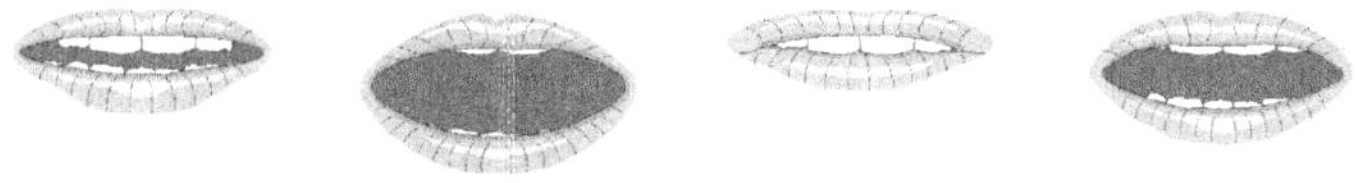

C

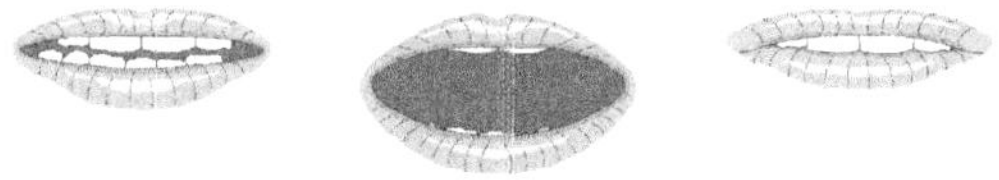

D

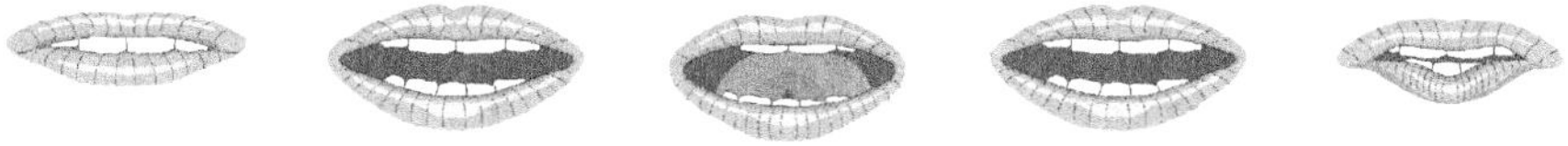

Highlight the voiced and unvoiced F/V sounds in the following text:

The feverfew plant is a member of the daisy family.
It is widely distributed throughout Europe North America and Australia.

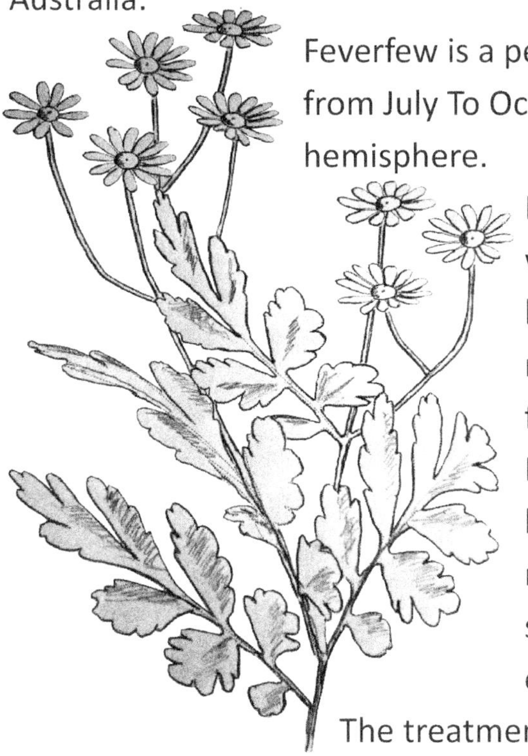

Feverfew is a perennial plant that flowers from July To October in the Northern hemisphere.

In ancient times feverfew was used to treat fevers but experiments in more recent time have not found it to be effective. Nowadays feverfew is believed to help prevent migraines and several studies suggest that it is effective for that purpose.

The treatment tried out by migraine sufferers was to eat two or three fresh leaves daily. Alternatively feverfew supplements can be obtained from health food shops.

The clues to the word puzzle are written in phonetic text – can you find all the words?

C.a.r.u.v.a.n.	F.i.sh.	R.e.f.ew.j.	V.ah.z.
C.er.f.ew.	F.r.ow.n.	R.u.f.	V.i.l.i.j.
F.ay.s.	F.ew.t.ure.	T.u.f.	F.e.ch.
F.r.ay.z.	V.a.l.ew.	S.t.u.f.i.ng.	F.a.sh.u.n.
F.oh.t.u.g.r.ah.f.			

	A	B	C	D	E	F	G	H	I	J
1	P	A	R	G	F	R	A	C	S	E
2	H	F	E	O	I	A	H	R	A	E
3	H	C	T	T	S	V	P	T	U	R
4	F	P	H	O	H	A	N	U	O	R
5	A	V	F	R	C	U	R	F	U	G
6	C	A	V	O	W	N	F	E	W	H
7	E	L	A	F	A	S	H	I	O	N
8	E	U	S	R	S	T	U	T	O	U
9	I	V	E	E	F	U	F	F	H	G
10	L	L	A	G	E	G	E	I	N	G

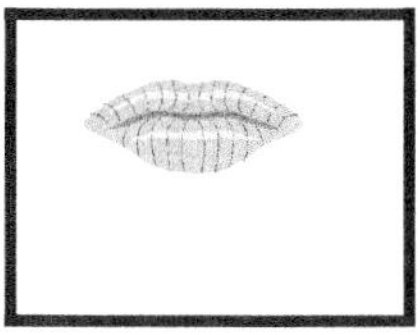

9. Lip Shape W

accompanies Q and W sounds

The W sound is made when the lips are tightly closed and puckered.

Lip shape M　**Lip shape W**　**Lip shape OO**　**Lip shape R**

The sound itself comes from the nose as does the M sound which can be made continuously so long as one has breath. With the W sound there is an additional internal and invisible constriction so that it is difficult to hold the sound continuously. The loudest part comes as the lips part at the end, and the sound, having been bottled up, bursts out from the parted lips as we say W...U.

The lip reader sees the closed and puckered lips to read the W while the release at the end gets absorbed into the vowel that follows.

When the Q sound is made, it's really two sounds, a K and a W. The K part merges with whatever precedes the W to become more or less invisible. So in lip reading we tend to put Q and W together.

Lip shape W finds its proper place at the beginning of words:

Quote	Wish	Waste	Quid	Want	Winter
Quickly	Wise	Wide	Wool	Worth	Word

Wish **W** **I** **SH**

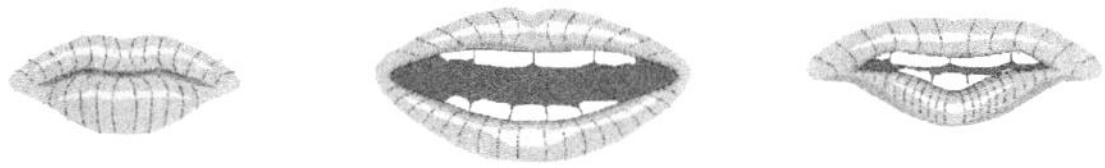

Lip shape W only fits into the middle of words in very specific circumstances.

Squeak	Swank	Swell	Swallow	Tweet
Twice	Twinkle	Twaddle	Dwelling	Tweezers

Tweet **T** **W** **EE** **T**

When W follows a vowel lip shape OO is often substituted:

Shower	Mower	Crown	Flower	Bellowing
Down	Growing	Towing	Towel	Borrowed

The written W at the end of words usually becomes the OO lip shape:

Bow	Show	Flow	Dough	New
Stew	Brew	Now	How	Allow

Flow F L O W

Class practice phrases:

Quick on the draw	Well wisher
Man and wife	Quick brew up
Crown Jewels	Town crier
Brown as a berry	Long frown
Blustery shower	Wednesday week
Stone wall	Show business
Borrowed time	Mow down

--------------------------------**Activities:**--------------------------------

Use a mirror to determine which of the following words uses lip shape W and which uses lip shape OO:

Twine	Newt	Lower	Shower	Swift
Swan	Crowd	Dwelling	Snowing	Newest

The lip-shape pictures show the first lip-shape seen when each word listed below is spoken:

WORTH SWELL MOW LOWER

Using a mirror to watch your own lips as you say the words, can you match the words on the list to the correct lip-shapes?

A 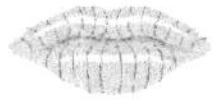 B 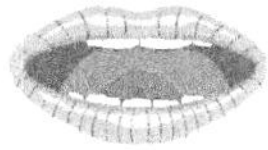 C 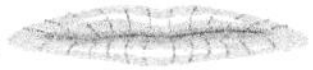 D 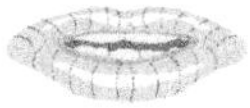

Highlight all the occurrences of lip shape W in the text:

Can you find words where lip shape W is used but it is not spelled with a W.
Can you find words that contain the letter W but where lip shape OO is used instead.

A wolf was on the loose near the Zoo after breaking through a wire fence and vanishing into the woods.

Police cordoned off a wide area of undergrowth while they searched for the missing wolf.

The alarm was raised when five wolves escaped through a damaged fence while a sixth wolf stayed behind.

All but one were accounted for but two had to be shot dead.

One of the wolves returned of its own accord another was recaptured.

The remaining wolf was thought to be sheltering in the nearby woods.

Complete the word puzzle:

The clues are in phonetic text.

Q.oh.t.	W.ay.s.t.	W.i.n.t.er.	B.e.l.oh.i.ng.
Q.i.k.l.ee.	W.er.th.	S.w.o.l.oh.	T.w.ee.z.er.z.
T.w.i.n.k.l.	B.o.r.oh.d.	F.l.ow.er.	D.w.e.l.i.ng.
W.i.sh.	S.q.ee.k.	T.oh.i.ng.	

	A	*B*	*C*	*D*	*E*	*F*	*G*	*H*	*I*	*J*
1	T	E	D	E	I	C	S	F	L	O
2	S	A	W	W	U	K	W	A	L	W
3	I	N	R	O	Q	L	S	H	L	E
4	W	G	R	O	B	Y	I	W	O	R
5	O	E	Z	E	R	S	W	Q	U	O
6	T	E	W	I	N	T	E	R	E	T
7	D	W	T	I	N	G	E	H	I	W
8	W	E	L	L	N	K	L	T	N	O
9	U	E	A	W	I	W	O	R	G	L
10	Q	S	K	T	N	O	W	B	E	L

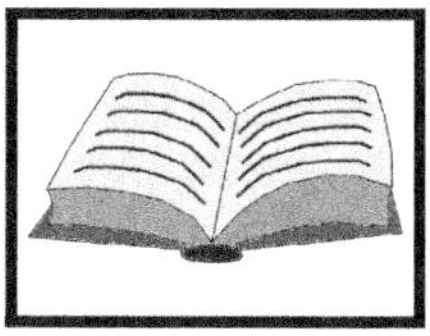

10. Lip shape text

writing text as a list of lip shapes

Below are three words set out as sequences of lip-shapes the lip reader would see as they are spoken – can you work out what those words are?

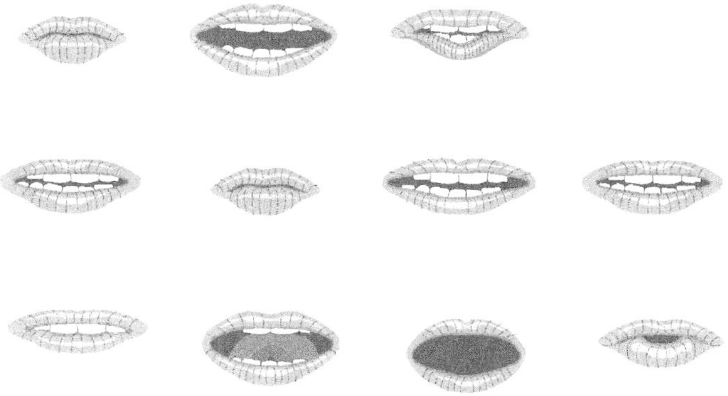

Unless you are very familiar with lip-shapes it is quite difficult to work out what the words are. And indeed when you are lip-reading you haven't got the time to puzzle it out. Fortunately, when you lip read for real, there is movement and you have other clues to go on and the process becomes automatic.

In the learning situation it becomes convenient to use a half-way house. Lip shapes have names, and if we can use the names for some of our activities we can practise separately some of the component parts that go to make up the process of lip reading.

*So here are the same words listed above but written as sequences of **lip shape names:***

W.I.J.   T.W.EE.T.   V.L.O.OO.

*Here they are again as **sounds:***

W.I.SH.   T.W.EE.T.   F.L.OH.

*And now as **normal spelling:***

WISH   TWEET   FLOW

This middle way is called lip shape text and is a way of writing down a copy of what the lips are doing as they speak.

You can see that there is a natural progression from the lip shape sequence to the lip-shape text to phonetic text to the spelling as we know it.

Neither interpreting a series of lip shape pictures nor reading lip shape text is the same as actual lip reading but they do give the opportunity to practise separately the various skills that collectively make up lip reading.

Here is another sequence of lip shapes:

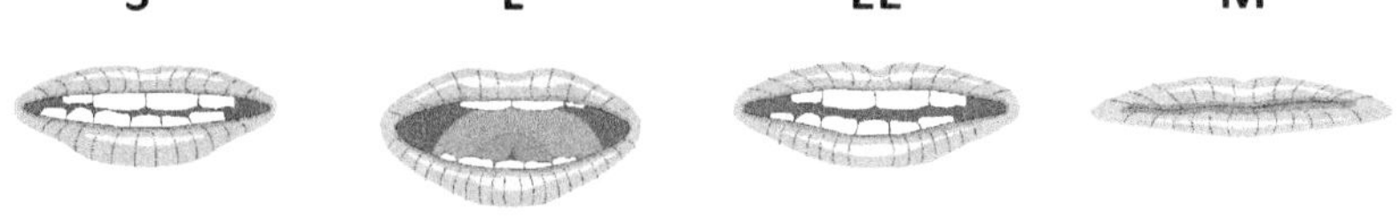
S
L
EE
M

Written as lip shape text it becomes: s.l.ee.m

What does this sequence say? It looks like "sleem", but there's no such word! We already know that individual lip shapes can accompany a number of different sounds – in this case lip shape M could indicate either a "M" or a "P" or a "B". The word is of course "Sleep". And if the lip reader had spotted this sequence in a sentence saying "I went to 'sleem' while watching the television" it would have been very obvious what the correct interpretation was.

But things are not always that easy and lip shape M is not the only lip shape that has multiple interpretations. The table below contains the complete set. It is reproduced in appendix A5 for easy reference.

Lip shape text is simply a shortened version of phonetic text.

The matter of determining the correct meaning from a number of alternatives is part and parcel of the lip reader's skill. The purpose of reading lip shape text is to give us practice in making those choices at lip reading speed without having, at the same time, to recognize all the various lip shapes.

Lip shape text is to the student of lip reading what sheet music is to the musician.

Basic Lip Shape Text

Lip shape	Sound(s)	Lip shape	Sound(s)
A	A, AH	**O**	O
AIR	AIR	**OH**	OH
AY	AY	**OI**	OI
E	E	**OO**	OO
EAR	EAR	**OW**	OW
EE	EE	**R**	R
ER	ER	**S**	S, X, Z
EW	EW	**T**	T, D, N
I	I	**TH**	TH
IA	IA	**U**	U
II	II	**URE**	URE
J	J, CH, SH, ZH	**UU**	UU, AW
K	K, C, G, H	**V**	V, F
L	L	**W**	W, Q
M	M, P, B	**Y**	Y
NG	NG		

-------------------------------Activities:--------------------------------

Here are two sets of words, one in conventional English spelling the other as lip shape text – match the normally spelled words to their equivalent lip shape versions:

Normally spelled words:

Barter *Butter* *Frequent* *Harbour*
Master *Parlour* *Pastry* *Prudent*
Puddle *Putty* *Quibbling* *Simple*
Wafer *Wager* *Willing*

Lip shape words:

W.i.l.i.ng.	*S.i.m.m.l.*	*K.a.m.er.*	*W.ay.j.er.*
V.r.ee.w.t.t.	*M.r.ew.t.u.t.t.*	*M.u.t.l.*	*M.u.t.er.*
M.a.s.t.er.	*M.a.t.er*	*M.a.l.er.*	*M.u.t.ee.*
M.ay.s.t.r.ee.	*W.i.m.l.i.ng.*	*W.ay.v.er*	

The clues to the word puzzle are in lip shape text – find the English spelled equivalent in the word puzzle:

M.l.ee.s.m.uu.t.	M.uu.t.i.ng.	V.l.ay.v.er.s.	K.o.l.i.t.ay.
M.er.m.l.	K.oh.m.v.uu.l.	K.r.u.m.m.l.	W.e.t.i.ng.
M.er.v.e.k.t.	S.l.oh.m.i.ng.	J.oi.s.	W.i.n.t.
L.o.s.t.	T.r.i.ng.k.	L.ii.t.	W.o.s.m.

	A	*B*	*C*	*D*	*E*	*F*	*G*	*H*	*I*	*J*
1	S	R	U	O	V	C	M	B	L	E
2	D	D	I	L	A	R	U	K	N	I
3	U	G	N	F	P	O	C	E	M	R
4	P	L	U	H	O	L	I	N	A	D
5	P	G	F	E	P	P	L	I	D	A
6	U	N	I	D	D	E	O	H	T	Y
7	R	P	L	E	E	R	F	E	C	G
8	C	I	N	D	W	L	O	P	I	N
9	H	W	L	I	G	S	P	S	A	W
10	O	I	C	E	H	T	L	O	S	T

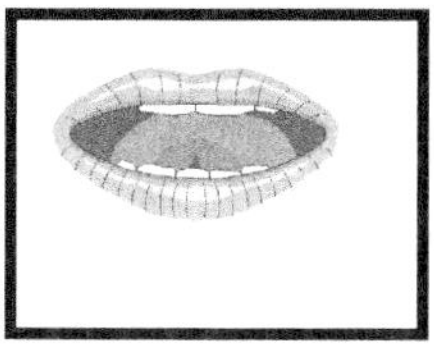

11. Lip Shape L

accompanies the L sound

Description of lip shape L:
It is not really a lip shape because the action takes place inside the mouth.

Visible evidence of the L sound is when you see the underside of the tongue as it goes up to the roof of the mouth.

This is different from TH when you see the edge of the tongue showing between the teeth.

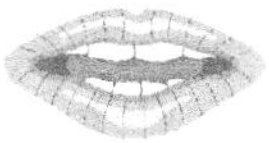

Lip shape TH

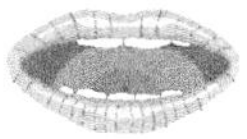

Lip shape L

It is also different from E when the tongue comes forwards but remains at the bottom of the mouth – in this case we see the upper surface of the tongue.

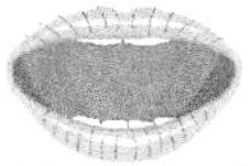

Lip shape E

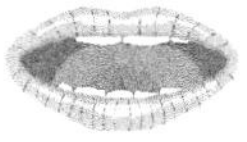

Lip shape L

Watch the tongue move as these words are spoken:
Lake Lair Left Led – (this is the L to E transition).

Watch and compare:

Left/Theft	Low/Though	Link/Think	Tile/Tithe
Will/With	Lot/Not	Let/Net	Line/Nine
Lest/Nest	Lock/Knock	Low/Know	Light/Night

L is difficult to see with sounds like EE, S and T - (it is hidden behind the teeth).

Check this is the case:

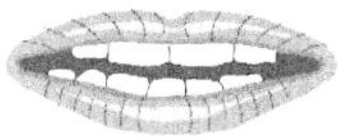

Seal	Steal	Sleep	Silver
Silk	Feel	Kettle	Little
Meal	Fill	Leave	

L is difficult to see with vowels like OO and AW - (it is in the dark cavity formed when the lips come forward).

Check this is the case:

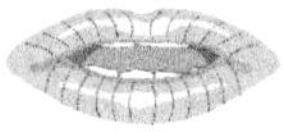

Tool	Fool	Rule	Mule
School	Fall	Wall	Tall
Small	Careful		

Class practice phrases:

A Light work
B A living wage
C A level playing field
C Silver lining
D Jolly good
E Jolly careful
F College place
G Travelling salesman
H Travel card
I Large as life
J Earn a living
K Lost for words
L Silver spoon
M Flight of fancy
N Silver collection
O College work
P Smooth as silk
Q A silky texture
R Labour of love
S University challenge

--------------------------------Activities:--------------------------------

Using a mirror to watch your own lips match the words on the list to the correct lip-shapes?

The lip-shape pictures show the first lip-shape seen when the names below are spoken:

FELICITY, JILL, LARRY, OLIVER, PAUL, RACHAEL, SYLVIA, WILLIAM

A 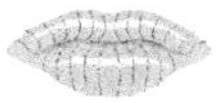 B 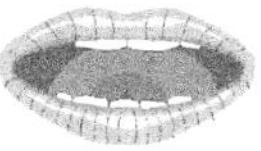 C 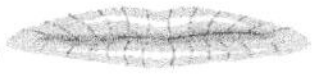 D 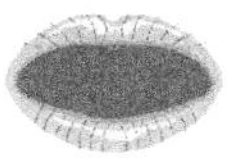

E 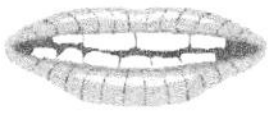 F 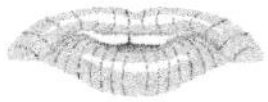 G 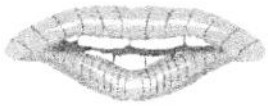 H 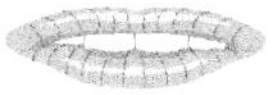

Using the table of consonant look-alikes work out what the lip shape text below is saying:

A U l.e.v.l m.l.ay.i.ng v.ee.l.t.

B Y.oo.n.i.v.er.s.i.t.ee j.a.l.e.n.j.

C L.i.m r.ee.t.i.ng i.s t.i.v.i.k.u.l.t i.v m.ee.m.l j.ow.t.

D L.i.m r.ee.t.i.ng i.s m.o.s.i.m.l oh.n.l.ee w.e.n m.ee.m.l v.ay.s y.oo.

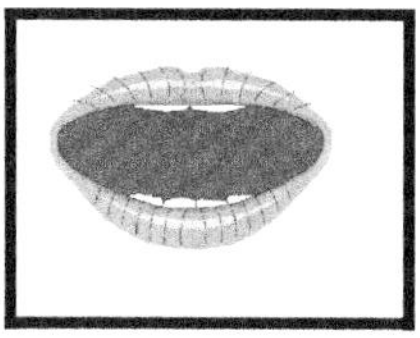

12. Lip Shape A

accompanies A (hat), AH (heart, OW1 and II1 sounds

E A and AH all share very similar lip shapes but the tongue is placed differently in each case:

E **A** **AH**

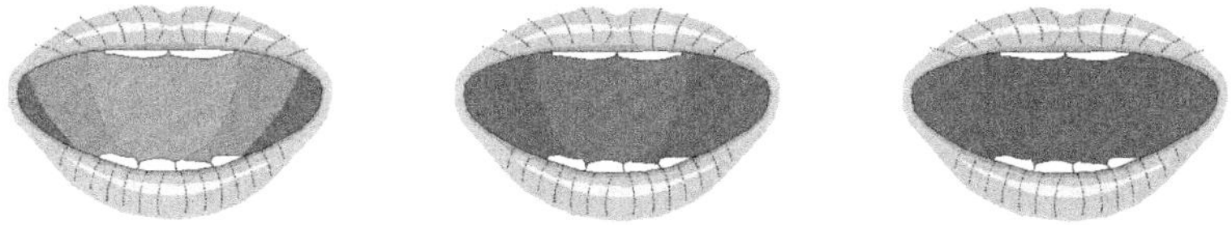

There is a slight visual difference between A and AH but it is very difficult to notice so they are grouped together as one lip shape.

Compare:

Den/Dan/Darn	Beg/Bag/Bark
Better/Batter/Barter	Head/Hat/Heart
Pet/Pat/Part	Letter/Ladder/Larder

Watch the lips as these words are spoken:

Market	Chance	Crab	Apple
Fast	Hand	Party	Wax
Rapid	Tramp	Land	Panic
Grand	Can	Thank	Gardens

Class practice phrases:

A. Taking part
B. Last chance
C. Land of the free
D. As quick as you can
E. First past the post
F. Garden party
G. Panic attack
H. Common market
I. Crab apple tree
J. Grand design
K. Hand over hand
L. He who laughs last
M. Part and parcel
N. Cash in the bank

-------------------------------Activities:-------------------------------

Match the words to the correct lip-shapes?

The lip-shape pictures show the first lip-shape seen when the following words are spoken:

Apple, Chance, Fast, Land, Rapid, Task, Thank, Wax

A 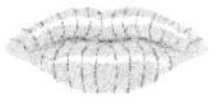

B 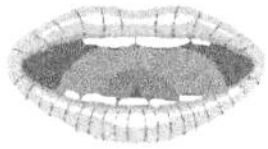

C 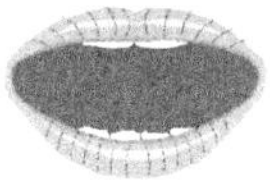

D 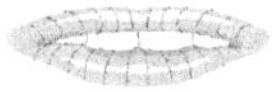

E 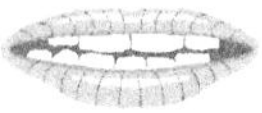

F 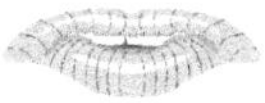

G 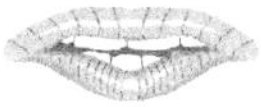

H 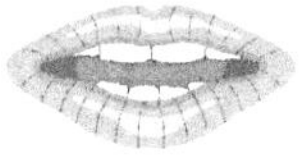

The clues for the word puzzle are in lip shape text – all are words already used in this lesson:

L.ah.j.er.	R.ay.l.w.ay.	K.ay.m.	K.l.ah.s.
T.ay.s.	M.ah.k.e.t.	J.ah.t.s.	K.r.a.m.
A.m.l.	M.ah.s.t.	K.a.t.t.	M.ah.t.ee.
M.ah.t.	R.a.m.i.t.	T.r.a.m.m.	M.a.t.i.k.
K.r.a.t.t.	K.a.t.	K.ah.t.e.t.s.	R.ah.th.er.

	A	*B*	*C*	*D*	*E*	*F*	*G*	*H*	*I*	*J*
1	G	E	R	R	A	Y	P	I	D	S
2	R	P	D	A	W	Y	A	R	E	N
3	A	M	N	I	L	T	C	A	M	E
4	L	A	A	H	A	R	G	A	R	D
5	T	R	S	D	P	S	S	A	L	C
6	D	A	Y	N	G	P	A	N	I	C
7	A	S	T	A	R	H	A	N	C	E
8	P	A	C	C	T	C	R	T	A	R
9	E	P	A	R	R	A	E	H	M	A
10	L	P	N	A	B	P	T	E	K	R

Highlight all the occurrences of lip shape A (A and AH) in the following text:

A very unusual property came onto the market in Cornwall in 2015.

It was an old railway carriage dating from the reign of Queen Victoria and the early days of the steam railways.

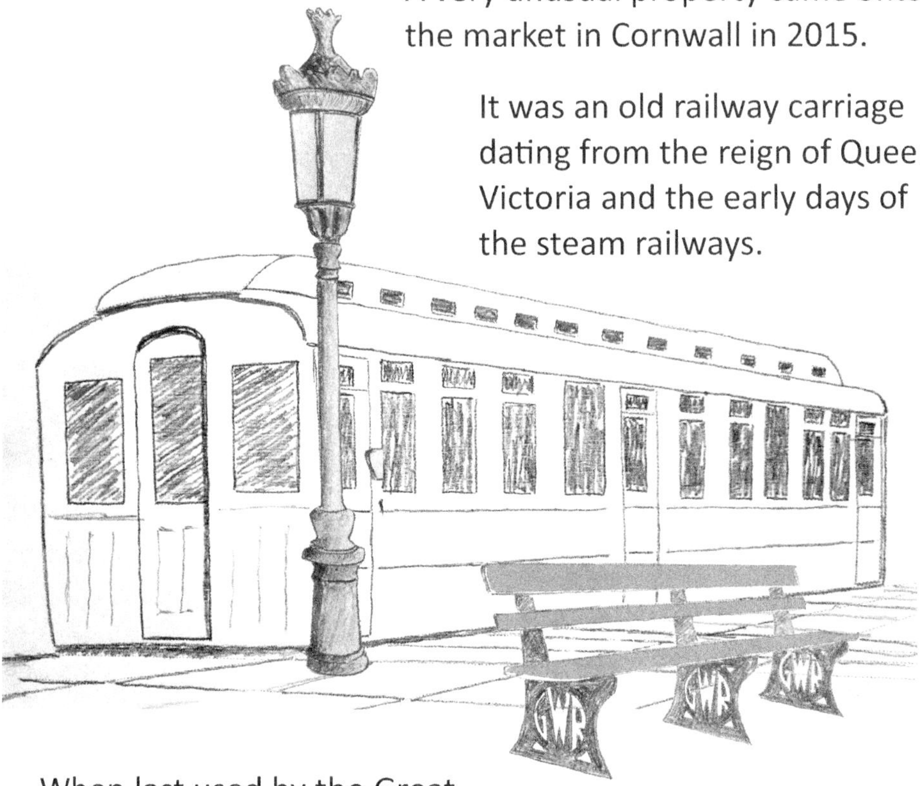
GWR
GWR
GWR

When last used by the Great Western Railway it was a third class carriage.

But restored to its original design by a later owner it is now a rather novel pair of bedrooms and part of a larger bungalow that has been built around it and decorated to look like a Victorian railway station.

(Remember that lip shape A is not the same as AY)

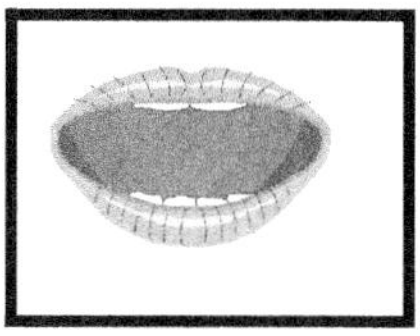

13. Lip Shape E

accompanies E (tent), AIR1 (care) and AY1 (hay) sounds

Lip shape E is similar to lip shape A but can be distinguished from it by the position of the tongue.

When we say E the tongue is pushed forward and placed behind the lower teeth. When we say A the tongue is further back and is less easy to see.

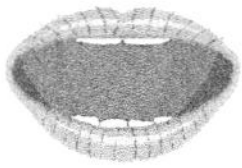

E

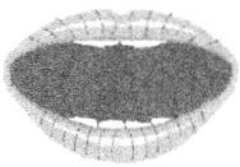

A

See the difference:

Ten/Ton/Tin/Tan	Guest/Gust
Ben/Bun/Bean/Bin/Ban	Medal/Muddle/Middle/Poodle

Observe the lips as these words are spoken:

Entry	Effort	Escape	Elephant	Exercise
Any	Enough	Endorse	Edit	Edge

Class practice phrases:

A. Ever decreasing circles
B. Lemon marmalade
C. Leicester city
D. Better price
E. Heading for victory
F. Credit rating
G. Holiday let
H. Bread and butter
I. Evergreen bush
J. Silver shred marmalade
K. Incredible price
L. Bread pudding
M. Yellow fever
N. Every man for himself
O. Post a letter
P. Off to bed

--------------------------------Activities:--------------------------------

Mirror work – observe the difference:

Beg	Bag	Bark
Mesh	Mash	Marsh
Led	Lad	Lard

Change the words in capitals for look-alike words so that the phrases make sense:

A NEST of strength
WET the chips are down
DEAD green bottles
TENTED pride
Paying the REND
Being LET astray
FEN up to the teeth
A DEBT of thieves
At a TENTER age
Pitching a DENT
Off to PEN

Highlight the "E" sounds in the following text:

There are three species of elephant in the world
They are the Asian elephant, the African bush elephant and the African forest elephant
Only the Asian elephant has been domesticated
It can be trained to do many kinds of work
The two African species have not been domesticated
The cows live in family groups with their young
They are led by the dominant cow
The bulls, once they have matured, leave the herd
They live alone and meet the cows only for breeding
African elephant numbers are falling due to poaching
Poachers kill the elephants to obtain their tusks

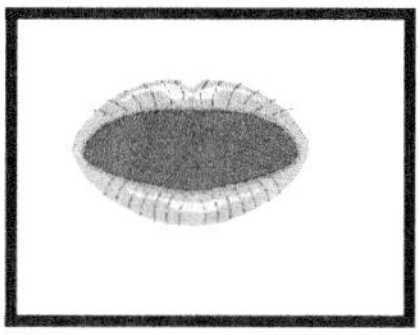

14. Lip Shape O

accompanies O and OH1 sounds

Lip shape O is rounded, the teeth are not prominent and the tongue is not seen.

The obvious characteristic is a dark cavity.

Lip shape O is smaller than lip shapes A and U but larger than lip shapes UU and OO.

Compare lip shape O with others:

	A	U	O	UU	OO
eg.	bag	bug	bog	book	pool

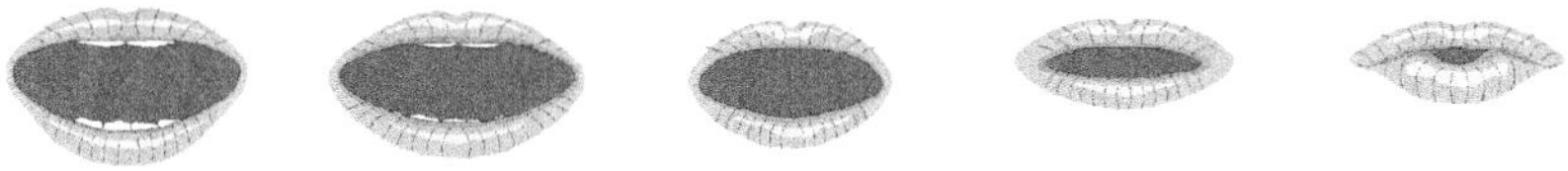

Observe how these words look on the lips:

O at the start of the word:

Odd	Office	Offer	Object	Oxford
On	Operation	Olive	Ostrich	Otter
Obscure	Offence	Offer	Oppose	Honour

O in the middle of the word:

Cross	Toss	From	Chop	Lost
Trodden	Shot	Fox	Trot	Gloucester
Knob	Hob	Lob	Lorry	Quad

Compare:

Loss/Loose Stop/Steep

Class practice phrases:

A. Clock watching
B. Dream topping
C. Shocking story
D. Daylight robbery
E. Office job
F. Stop the rot
G. Climb to the top
H. Cross words
I. Well trodden
J. Win the lottery
K. Top dog
L. Good offer
M. Shop till you drop
N. Shot in the dark

--------------------------------Activities:--------------------------------

Match the words to the correct lip-shapes

The lip-shape pictures show the first lip-shape seen when the following words are spoken:

Chop, Frog, Long, Mop, Rubber, Stop, Those, Whopper

A 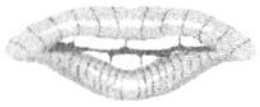 B 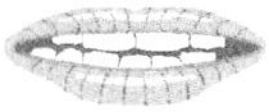 C 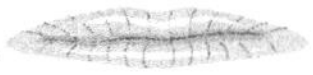 D 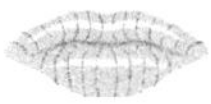

E 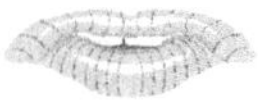 F 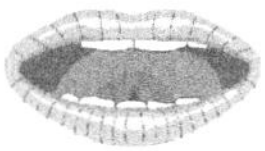 G 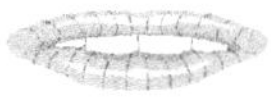 H 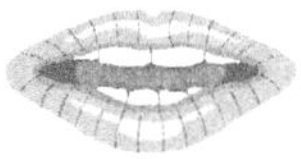

The clues to the word puzzle are words used above but are in lip shape text – can you complete the puzzle?

K.r.o.s.	V.r.o.m.	K.o.m.	O.t.er.
J.o.m.	L.o.r.ee.	L.o.t.er.ee.	O.m.s.k.ure.
O.v.e.n.s.	O.v.er.	O.v.i.s.	O.l.i.v.
O.m.er.ay.j.u.t.	O.m.oh.s.	R.o.m.er.ee.	
J.o.k.i.ng.	T.r.o.t.e.t.		

	A	B	C	D	E	F	G	H	I	J
1	U	R	Y	R	R	H	O	O	S	E
2	O	H	S	L	O	O	P	P	P	E
3	N	O	H	O	C	B	E	O	O	C
4	L	O	Y	R	K	A	R	F	F	I
5	O	T	T	E	I	T	S	S	O	L
6	F	F	O	G	N	I	O	O	J	I
7	M	E	B	S	D	E	N	R	O	V
8	O	N	U	C	D	N	R	C	B	E
9	R	C	R	R	O	F	E	B	B	E
10	F	E	E	T	O	F	R	O	Y	R

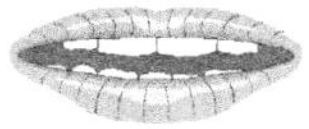

15. Lip Shape K

accompanies C, G, H and K sounds

Lip shape K is very variable and is sometimes classed as an invisible - there is certainly a lip shape there every time one of the consonants is spoken but because the sound can be made with almost any open lip shape, every time it is spoken, the accompanying lip shape is similar to the vowel which precedes or follows it. The presence of the sound is generally only discerned from the fact that there is a slight delay between the vowel and consonant.

Compare:

At/act	Ass/axe	Air/care	Crate/rate
Park/par		Heart/art	Litter/glitter

C G H words to observe:

Carry	Go	High	Catch	Girl
Home	King	Grated	Track	Quay
Elk	Brag	Hit	Back	Picnic
Begin	Hall	History	Garden	Emigrate
Gathers	Signal	Harvest		

These words are hard to tell apart

Cow/How	Coast/Ghost/Host
Card/Guard/Hard	Kate/Gate/Hate
Calm/Harm	Kite/Height
Curl/Girl/Hurl	Crab/Cram/Grab

- but context helps to show which word is being spoken.

Class practice phrases:

A. Grab some lunch
B. Crazy idea
C. Practical joke
D. Clever child
E. Sticky wicket
F. Comfortable seat
G. Cost of living
H. Ice cream cornet
I. Kind hearted man
J. Christmas cake
K. Garden gate
L. Credit card

------------------------------**Activities:**------------------------------

Use a mirror to match the words to the correct lip-shapes

The lip-shape pictures show the first lip-shape seen when the following words are spoken:
Cat, Clever, Cook, Cool, Cot, Cruel, Cuddle, Kettle:

A 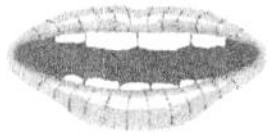 B 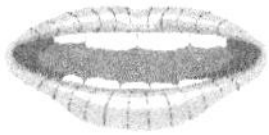 C 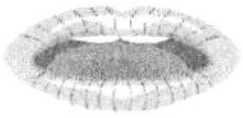 D 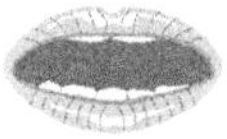

E 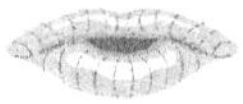 F 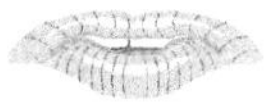 G 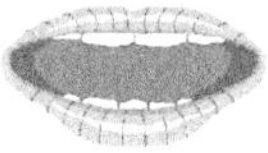 H 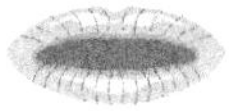

Solve the word puzzle with words used in this lesson:

The clues are lip shape text:

M.a.k.	K.ah.m.	K.a.r.ee.	K.a.j.
K.r.i.s.m.us	K.l.e.v.er.	K.aw.t.i.t.	K.r.ay.s.ee.
K.r.ee.m.	K.r.e.t.i.t.	K.ah.t.e.t.	K.a.th.er.
K.l.ee.m.	K.l.i.t.er.s.	K.r.ay.t.i.t.	K.ay.s.t.
K.ow.	S.t.i.k.ee.		

	A	B	C	D	E	F	G	H	I	J
1	R	E	A	M	Y	G	D	R	S	H
2	C	L	M	C	Z	R	E	E	C	C
3	C	A	G	R	A	A	T	T	A	T
4	H	T	A	N	G	A	G	T	R	E
5	E	R	Y	E	D	R	L	I	C	D
6	A	R	R	S	T	I	C	K	T	I
7	C	R	L	E	A	M	H	Y	C	K
8	V	E	G	E	T	S	A	S	A	C
9	E	H	O	N	C	T	M	A	B	H
10	L	C	W	R	O	E	T	S	I	R

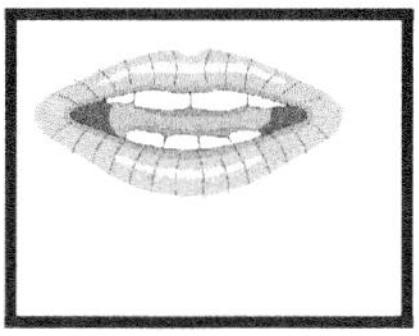

16. Lip Shape TH

accompanies the TH sound

The TH sound is made when the tongue is between the parted teeth. Both tongue and teeth are necessary to make this sound. The tongue and teeth in their relative positions are fairly easy to see though the movement is fast.

In some people the tongue overshoots the teeth and becomes very visible in others it only just reaches the teeth and is less easy to see.

The TH sound can be unvoiced and hard to hear as in words like Thick and Thorn or it can be voiced and easier to hear in words like Bathe (compare Bath and Bathe to hear the difference).

To the lip reader the two TH lip shapes are the same.

Unvoiced TH words:

Thing	Thank	Thought	Through	Both
Teeth	Thin	Thorough	Nothing	Bath

Voiced TH words:

The	This	Then	Clothes	With
Weather	Bother	Other	Them	Bathe

Compare the lip shapes as these words are spoken:

Thank/Bank	Throw/Low	Thought/Fought
Think/Link/Pink	With/Will/Win	Thick/Wick/Click

Compare the lip shapes:

Lip shape E | Lip shape L | Lip shape TH | Lip shape V

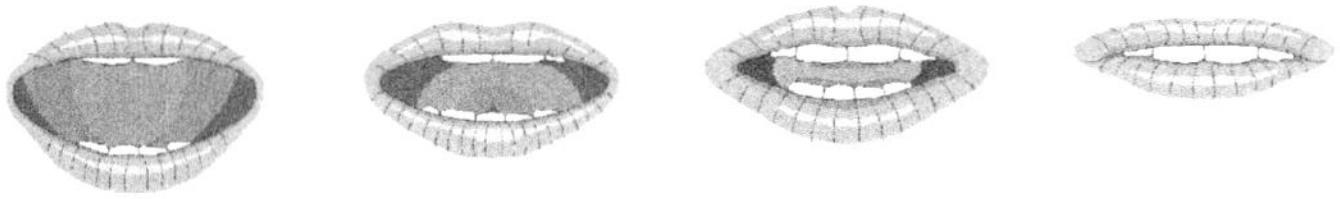

Class practice phrases:

A. Thick and thin
B. Cold weather
C. Great North Road
D. Rather good
E. Think about it
F. Needle and thread
G. This and that
H. Thought provoking
I. Weather station
J. Withheld information
K. Food for thought
L. Leather boots
M. Brother and sister
N. Next month

---------------------------------Activities:---------------------------------

Which words are these?

A. Looks like: **M O TH ER**

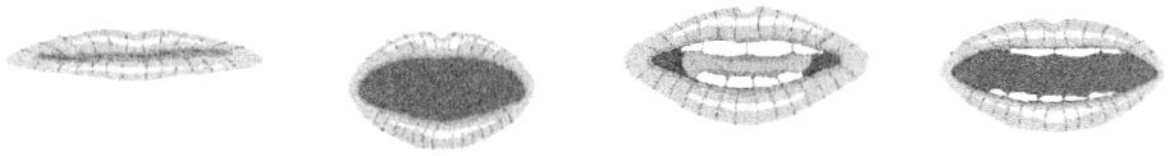

B. Looks like: **TH U R U**

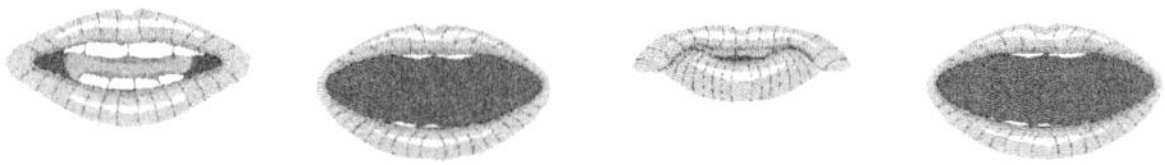

C. Looks like: **V AW TH**

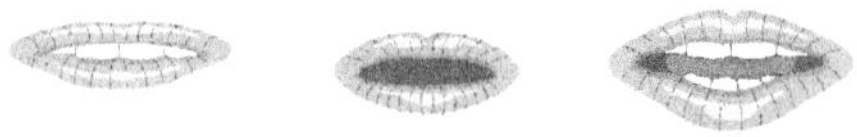

D. Looks like: **W E TH ER**

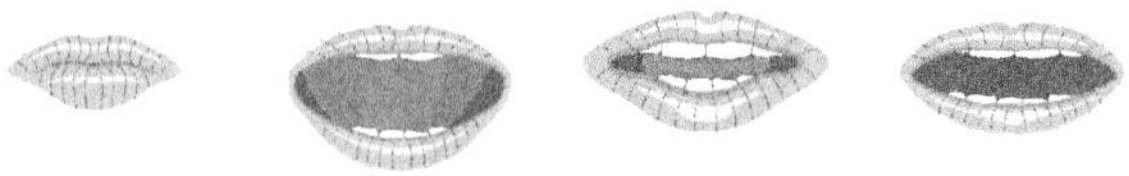

Solve the word puzzle with words used in this lesson:

The clues are in lip shape text:

M.ah.th.	M.ay.th.	M.oh.th.	K.l.oh.th.s.
L.e.th.er.	M.u.t.th.	T.aw.th.	T.u.th.i.ng.
U.th.er.	R.ah.th.er.	T.ee.th.	TH.a.ng.k.
TH.a.t.	TH.e.m.	TH.i.k.	TH.u.r.u.
W.e.th.er.	W.i.th.		

	A	*B*	*C*	*D*	*E*	*F*	*G*	*H*	*I*	*J*
1	E	S	E	H	H	E	T	T	H	E
2	H	L	C	T	T	R	H	O	T	R
3	T	O	B	A	A	H	A	T	H	E
4	R	A	T	W	E	T	B	A	T	H
5	O	T	H	E	R	E	O	N	T	H
6	N	H	I	N	G	E	M	H	A	N
7	T	H	O	T	H	T	T	T	K	K
8	W	I	R	A	E	M	H	I	C	H
9	H	T	O	E	R	E	N	O	R	T
10	H	G	U	L	T	H	B	O	T	H

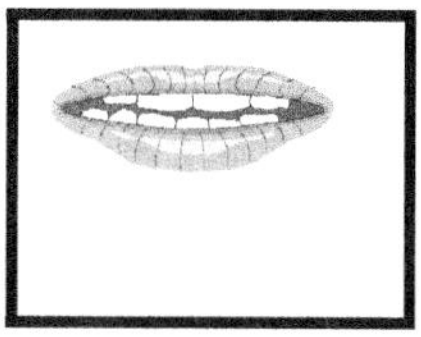

17. Lip Shape T

accompanies D, N and T sounds

Lip shape T is similar to lip shape S and they are difficult to tell apart.
There is a small visible difference in that with lip shape T the teeth are not so tightly clenched as with lip shape S

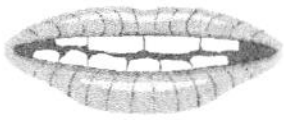

Lip shape S

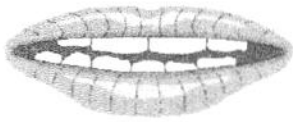

Lip shape T

The important differences that modify the sound to become S or T or D or N are behind the teeth and are unlikely to be spotted by the lip reader.

The lip reader needs to rely on other clues to distinguish between the two lip shapes.

Observe T D N at start of words:

Time	Did	Knock	Tries	Nobody	Treat
Dread	Title	Nought	Doll	Track	Never

Observe T D N in the middle of words:

Penny	Kettle	Monday	Ladle	Button	Cuddle
Undo	Anvil	Lantern	Fiddle	Antacid	Addition

Observe T D N at the end of words:

That	Hard	Crane	Loan	Cricket	Carpet
Paid	Ward	Freed	Great	Frown	Condition

Observe words where the N sound accompanies NG:

Anxious	Plank	Mangle	Frank	Junk	Link
Monkey	Rank	Extinct	Brink	Shrink	Function

Words that look similar

Till/Dill/Nil	Toll/Doll/Knoll	Tried/Dried
Latter/Ladder	Spatter/Spanner	Ton/Done/Nun
Flat/Flan	Moat/Mode/Moan	Dock/Knock

Class practice phrases:

A. Danger money
B. The devil's in the detail
C. Dry cleaning
D. Duty bound
E. National scandal
F. Never say die
G. Can't stop
H. Stop and start
I. Do or die
J. Never a dull word
K. Dark deed
L. Drink and drive
M. TV drama
N. Window shopping
O. Burnt fingers
P. Point of view

--------------------------------Activities:--------------------------------

Use a mirror to check how you say these words:

The lip-shape pictures show the first lip-shape seen when I say the words. How different are your lip shapes?:

TEETH

A 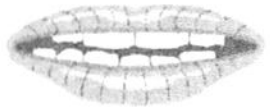

TERMINUS

B 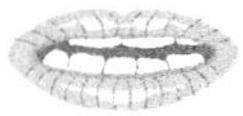

TOOTH

C 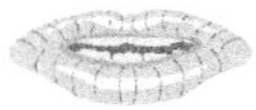

TOOK

D 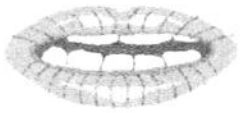

Exchange the words in capitals for look-alike words so that the text below makes sense

There are PENNY species of terrapin.

SUP live in the warmer BARNS of the United States in fresh or brackish water.

They HAT live in SEE water but DEED fresh water DO drink.

Fresh water is lighter than salt WARDER so in estuaries tends DO stay on the surface.

In such circumstances terrapins have BEAD seen to CUP to the surface to drink thus avoiding drinking the salty WARDER below the surface.

The female terrapin LACE her eggs in the spring and buries them under the sand.

She then goes MAC into the WARDER and does NOD return.

The eggs incubate and CADGE in the warm sand but the gender of the hatchlings is determined PIE the temperature OFF the sand INN which they incubate.

People sometimes HEAP terrapins as PENS. In the indoor aquarium their colour is GREED.

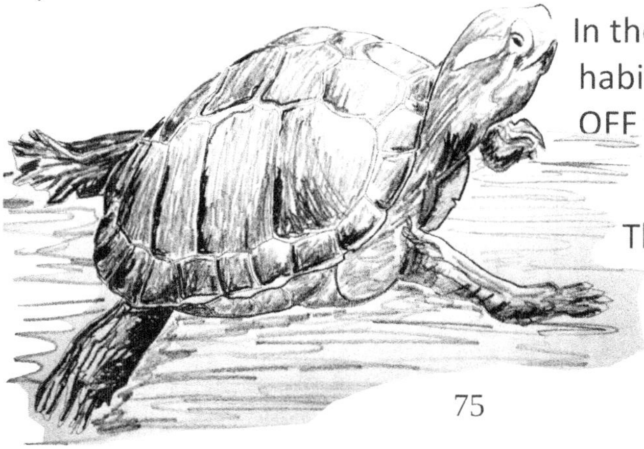

In the wild they have a habit of coming out OFF the water TWO lie in the SUD.

This BAKES them much darker in colour.

Complete the word puzzle – the clues are in lip shape text:

A.t.i.j.u.t.	K.o.t.t.i.j.t.	K.r.ay.t.	T.i.t.
E.s.t.i.ng.k.t.	M.e.t.ee.	M.a.ng.k.l.	T.r.ee.t.
K.ah.m.e.t.	T.o.l.	V.i.t.l.	T.r.e.t.
L.a.t.t.er.n.	V.u.ng.j.uu.t.	V.r.ow.t.	T.o.k.
T.oh.m.o.t.ee.			

	A	B	C	D	E	F	G	H	I	J
1	E	D	O	K	C	P	E	N	D	I
2	X	T	L	L	O	N	N	O	C	T
3	C	I	A	D	D	K	N	Y	D	I
4	A	N	C	T	I	T	I	D	I	O
5	R	P	N	T	F	I	O	N	F	N
6	T	R	E	A	T	D	A	D	U	N
7	F	R	O	E	L	D	E	R	D	C
8	N	T	W	N	O	B	O	C	N	T
9	A	E	R	N	N	M	D	R	O	I
10	L	E	L	G	N	A	Y	A	N	E

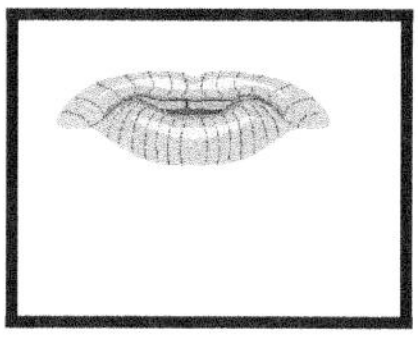

18. Lip Shape R

accompanies the R sound

Compare lip shape R with other similar lip shapes:

Y J R OO

With Lip shape R the lips are pushed forwards and puckered.
They are pushed forwards less than with lip shape J.
They are puckered less than with lip shape OO.

Observe lip shape R at the beginning of words:

Rack	Red	Roast	Rhyme	Really
Ribbon	Rest	Royal	Religion	Rainbow

Observe lip shape R in the middle of words:

Try	Burrow	Sorry	Worry	Narrow
Mirror	Turning	Bird	Clerk	Dearest

The R sound often gets lost (see Turning, Bird, Clerk) mainly at the end of words – it is usually replaced by the ER vowel:

Check whether Lip shape ER ends these words:

Laser	Wander	Flower	Rigour	Lower
Summer	Car	Mare	More	Share

With the R sound the teeth are parted.
With the J sound the teeth close as with the S sound.
Notice that J, Ch, Sh, and Zh sound similar to S.

With lip shape R the teeth cannot usually be seen.

Compare:

Rain/Chain/Stain	Rat/Chat/Sat	Marrow/Macho

Compare R with F

Rat/Fat	Rot/Font	Rook/Foot	Writ/Fit
Run/Fun	Real/Feel	Raid/Fade	Reed/Feed

Observe lip shape R preceded by other consonants:

Brain	Prick	Shrew	Thread	Trigger
Friday	Growing	Crack	Crime	Drink

Class practice phrases:

A. Wrong turning
B. Rover ticket
C. Sour cream
D. Really cheap
E. Sorry story
F. Practical Joke
G. Cradle to grave
H. Rise and Shine
I. River crossing
J. Rhyme and reason
K. Carried along
L. No problem
M. Profit and loss
N. Travel card

Notice in the above phrases that turning and card do not use lip shape R. Instead they use lip shape ER and lip shape A.

Rover, River and Sour end with lip shape ER.

--------------------------------**Activities:**--------------------------------

Which of these words do not end with lip shape ER?

Laser	Wander	Flower	Rigour	Lower
Summer	Car	Mare	More	Share

Match the words to the correct lip-shapes

The lip-shape pictures show the first lip-shape seen when the names of birds are spoken:

Albatross, Blackbird, Duck, Flamingo, Jay, Lark, Quail, Raven, Thrush, Wagtail

A 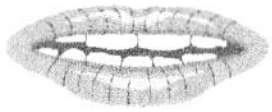 B 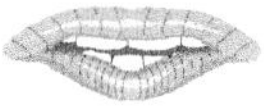 C 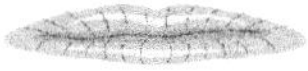 D 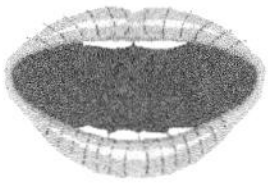

E 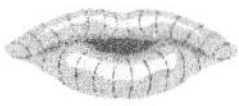 F 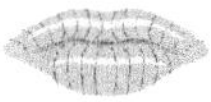 G 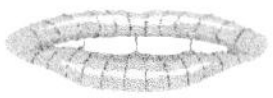 H 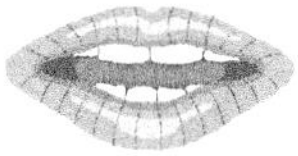

I 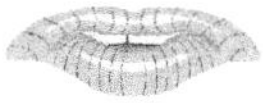 J 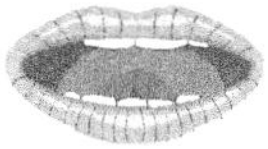

In the exercise below the words and phrases are given in lip shape text (lists of lip shapes).

Which of the above words are these?

M.er.t. M.u.r.oh. L.oh.er.

Which of the above phrases are these?

K.r.ay.t.l. t.oo. k.r.ay.v.
R.ii.m. a.n.t. r.ee.s.n.
M.r.a.k.t.l.k.l j.oh.k

Highlight the letter Rs in the following text that are spoken with lip shape R:

Driving to Mongolia

Three old school friends have set themselves the challenge of driving a Nisan Micra car from London To Mongolia to raise money for charity.

They will be taking part in the Mongol Rally over a distance of ten thousand miles.

The money raised will go to the Woking Hospice and also to a charity working to stop rainforest destruction.

The Mongol Rally sets out from Battersea Park in July.

The team have mapped out a rough route taking them through Turkey, Georgia, Azerbaijan, Kazakhstan and Russia. "We are trying not to plan too much as that's part of the fun."

Along the journey they will sleep in the car.

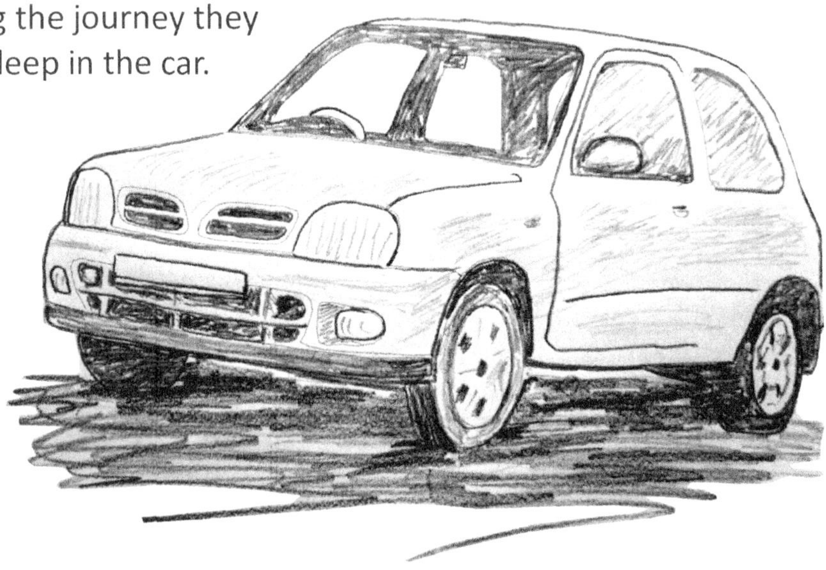

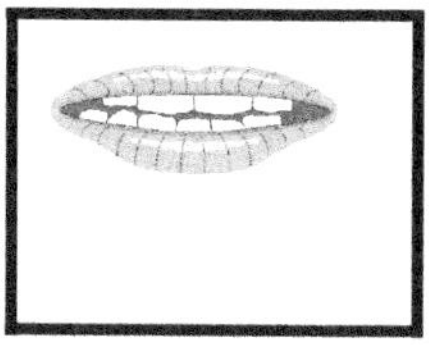

19. Lip Shape S

accompanies S, Z and X sounds

The S sound is made by blowing air between the clenched teeth and while making the sound the lips are pulled back revealing the teeth. The S and Z sounds are continuous and can be held for as long as one wants. The X is of short duration.

Lip shape S is also very similar to lip shape T and I find it difficult to tell them apart on the basis of lip shape alone. Instead I have to rely on context to distinguish which is being spoken.

Because the S sound is made at the teeth it does not depend on any particular arrangement of the lips. So long as the lips are parted so that the sound can come out the lips can be placed in a number of different ways without changing the sound (try it in front of a mirror). The effect of this is that for much of the time, when S, Z or X is spoken the lips are getting ready for the next sound. (Use a mirror to compare Sea and Zoo).

Class practice phrases:

A. Is that wise
B. Press report
C. New tricks
D. Taking possession
E. Extra chips
F. Nuisance calls
G. Sealed lips
H. Sudden movement
I. Excessive moisture
J. No flies on him
K. Fast food
L. Slippery surface
M. An exact science
N. Exact amount

--------------------------------**Activities:**--------------------------------

Look at S words in the mirror:

Single	Slime	Supper	Soon	Sock
Soup	Sudden	Razor	Mustard	Taxi
Facsimile	Wisdom	Rising	Exercise	Peas
Exchange	Peace	Nice	Fries	Twice

Match the words to the correct lip-shapes

The lip-shape pictures show the first lip-shape seen when the following words are spoken: **Seek, Soot, Soup.**

A 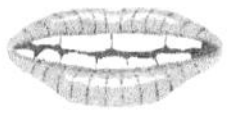 B 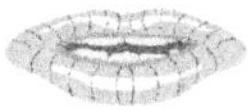 C 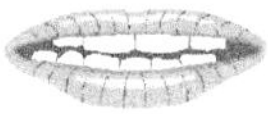

Underline instances of Lip shape S in the following text - Circle those that are sounded with a Z:

STENCILS

Stencils have been around for a very long time.

Pre historic stencil work has been found in Argentina.

Pre historic man's stencil was his hand .

He spat ink through it onto the cave wall .

Stencils can be made from most thin materials.

If they are strong enough they can be used many times.

It is not possible to make every shape using a simple stencil.

A stencil to print the shape of the letter O will fall apart.

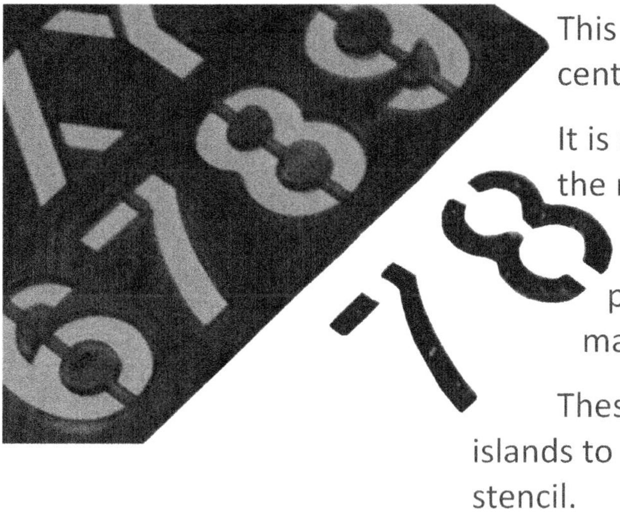

This is because the central part is an island.

It is not connected to the rest of the stencil.

To overcome this problem stencils are made with bridges.

These connect the islands to the rest of the stencil.

The bridges also prevent the ink from getting to the paper.

They leave gaps in the printed letters.

Complete the word puzzle – the clues are in lip shape text

M.a.s.i.m.u.m.	M.ee.s.	M.r.e.s.	R.ii.s.i.ng.
S.a.k.	S.ee.l.t.	S.i.ng.k.l.	S.ii.e.t.s.
S.l.i.m.er.ee.	S.o.k.	S.oo.m.	S.oo.t.
S.u.m.er.	S.u.t.	S.u.t.t.	T.a.s.ee.
S.i.k.t.uu.l.	T.ii.s.	T.r.i.k.s.	T.w.ii.s.

	A	B	C	D	E	F	G	H	I	J
1	E	D	O	K	C	P	E	N	D	I
2	X	T	L	L	O	N	N	O	C	T
3	C	I	A	D	D	K	N	Y	D	I
4	A	N	C	T	I	T	I	D	I	O
5	R	P	N	T	F	I	O	N	F	N
6	T	R	E	A	T	D	A	D	U	N
7	F	R	O	E	L	D	E	R	D	C
8	N	T	W	N	O	B	O	C	N	T
9	A	E	R	N	N	M	D	R	O	I
10	L	E	L	G	N	A	Y	A	N	E

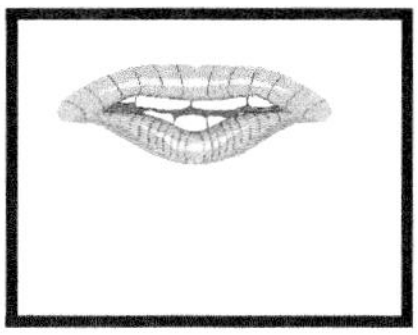

20. Lip Shape J

accompanies SH, CH, J and ZH sounds

The most prominent characteristic of lip shape J is the forward movement of the lips. It is easy to recognize.

Compare lip-shapes W, R and J:

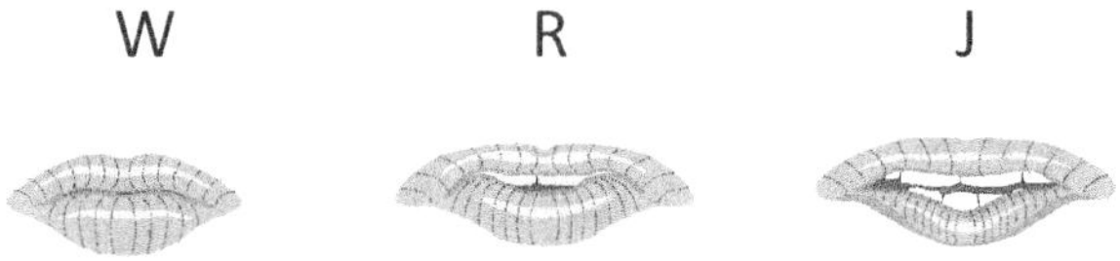
W
R
J

Observe the difference:

Whip	Rip	Ship
Wine	Ride	Shine

Lip-shape J accompanies the sounds CH as in "cherry", SH as in "shake", J as in "jam" and ZH as in "corrosion".

Observe lip shape J in these words:

Cheek	Shell	Just	Shake	Giraffe
Machine	Ancient	Ocean	Bachelor	Subject
Pleasure	Measure	Seizure	Collision	Garage
Edge	Batch	Blush	Wish	'Fridge

Observe words with similar lip-shapes:

Sheep/cheap/jeep
Mash/match/Madge
Catching/cashing/cadging

Class practice phrases:

A. Sugar free
B. Service charge
C. Treasure trove
D. Life of leisure
E. Bird watching
F. Nuclear fission
G. Just a minute
H. Cherry picking
I. Lock up garage
J. Pleasure park
K. Share and share alike
L. Precision engineering
M. Rough justice
N. Judge and jury

-------------------------------**Activities:**---------------------------------

Match up the words that will look similar on the lips:

Shop	Jane	Shane	Fletch	Jib	Ship
Chop	Jaw	Mash	Catch	Fledge	Flesh
Chain	Badge	Cash	Chore	Jean	Shore
Cheat	Cadge	Sheen	Match	Sheet	Chip

Highlight instances of lip shape J in this text:

Deep fried fish was introduced to England in the sixteenth century.
It was sold by Jewish refugees from the continent.
Fish and chips was a popular working class dish in the nineteenth century.
This was because trawl fishing produced a plentiful supply of fresh fish.
Deep fried chips first appeared in England in eighteen sixty.
They were sold in London by Joseph Malin a Jewish refugee.
During World War Two fish and chips was exempt from rationing.
But chip shop customers had to bring their own newspaper.
Traditional frying uses beef dripping or lard
however, vegetable oils, are often used instead.
American style French fries are thinner than English chips.
The larger surface area absorbs more fat.

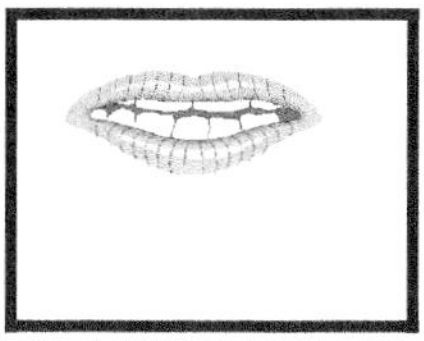

21. Lip Shape Y

accompanies URE and Y sounds

Lip shape Y is affected by the vowel that follows it and can be very variable.

Observe Lip shape Y at the start of words:

Yard	Yawn	You	Year	Yew
Yet	Yachts	Yellow	Youth	Yesterday
Usual	Young	Youthful	Europe	

Lip shape Y comes in the middle of words when the URE vowel is used.

Observe lip shape Y in the URE vowel:

Manure	Liquor	Fury	Curio	Secure

Frequently when the letter Y is used in spelling it is spoken using lip shape EE:

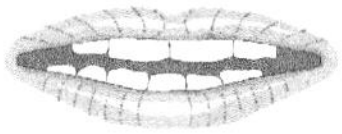

Check which lip shape accompanies the Y spelling:

Way	Carry	Wayside	Lay-by	Daytime
Easy	Yeast	Early	Yearly	Ladybird

Class practice phrases:

A. Help yourself
B. Yesterday's model
C. Young and beautiful
D. What a carry on
E. A lovely holiday
F. Fall by the wayside
G. Yorkshire pudding
H. Usual price
I. Stop worrying
J. Use the yard broom
K. Fast and furious
L. A secure loan

--------------------------------**Activities:**--------------------------------

The text below does not make sense. Exchange the words in capitals for look-alike words so that the text makes sense:

Yorkshire Pudding was described in eighteenth century cook books as TRIPPING pudding.
IN was served as the VERSED course of a PEEL to dampen the appetite.
This was so that NINERS would require less MEAN in the following COARSE.
It was a BUNNY saving practice INN households that were NOD so well OF.
In even poorer households there was TOW meat course and Yorkshire Pudding was the PEAL.
It was a MEATS of producing a nourishing MEEL using only dripping, FLOWER, milk and eggs.
IN is believed THAN its association with the county of Yorkshire was because OFF the availability of SHEEP coal.
Burning WHOLE produced the high temperatures required FOUR making Yorkshire Pudding WISH was often served with gravy.

Here are some of the above phrases written as lip shape text: – can you work out which they are?

K.e.l.m. y.aw.s.e.l.v.

W.o.t. u. k.a.r.ee. o.t.

Y.u.ng. a.t.t. m.ew.t.i.v.uu.l.

U. l.u.v.l.ee. k.o.l.i.t.ay.

EW.j.ew.u.l. m.r.ii.s.

V.ah.s.t. a.t.t. v.ure.ee.u.s.

Y.aw.k.j.u. m.uu.t.i.ng.

S.t.o.m. w.u.r.ee.i.ng.

The clues to the word puzzle are in lip shape text – can you solve the puzzle?

K.a.r.ee.	K.ure.ee.oh.	T.ay.t.ii.m.
ER.l.ee.	EE.s.ee.	V.ure.ee.
K.o.l.i.t.ay.	L.ay.t.ee.m.er.t.	L.u.v.l.ee.
S.e.k.ure.	EW.s.	EW.j.ew.u.l.
W.u.r.ee.i.ng.	Y.o.t.s.	Y.ah.t.
Y.er.	Y.ee.s.t.	Y.oo.th.v.uu.l.

	A	B	C	D	E	F	G	H	I	J
1	A	R	L	Y	E	M	I	F	U	R
2	E	Y	E	A	S	T	T	R	A	Y
3	D	A	Y	O	D	A	Y	U	E	Y
4	I	U	R	I	S	C	A	S	U	A
5	L	C	S	E	E	C	R	Y	A	L
6	O	H	U	T	S	U	R	Y	R	D
7	D	A	L	H	E	R	Y	O	U	T
8	Y	E	A	C	A	Y	G	U	F	H
9	B	D	S	L	Y	L	N	L	W	O
10	I	R	Y	E	V	O	I	Y	R	R

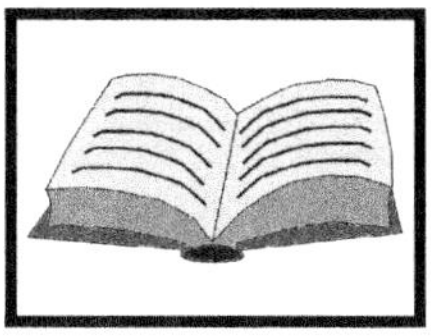

22. Sliding vowels 2

AIR, AY, IA, EAR, EW, II, OH, OI, OW, URE

Sliding vowels are different from the primary vowels listed in the appendix with the primary lip shapes. The sliding vowel sounds are made as the lips change their shape, passing through two or more lip shapes in quick succession.

Sometimes they are called double or multiple vowels.

There are ten sliding vowels to recognize when lip reading each with its own name. They are AIR, AY, IA, EAR, EW, II, OH, OI, OW and URE. Each one is described below and examples given.

***AIR** is formed from lip shape **E** followed by lip shape **ER**:*

AIR

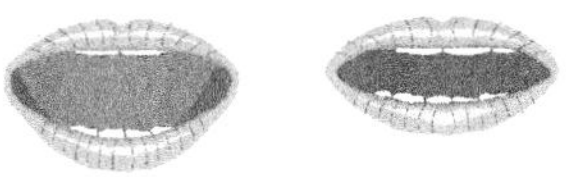

As in: Care, Stair, Pair, Dare, Chair and Hair

AY** is formed from lip shape **E** followed by lip shape **EE

AY

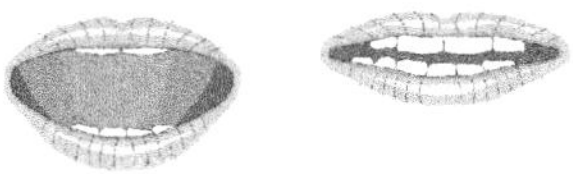

As in: Chain, Brain, Crane, Blame, Aid and Made.

***OW** is formed from lip shape **A** followed by lip shape **OO**:*

OW

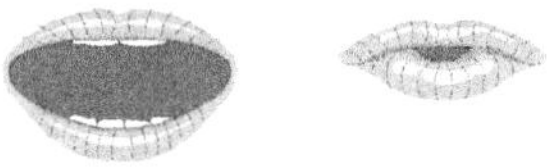

As in: Crowd, Frown, Hound, Shout, Loud, Trowel.

***IA** is formed from lip shape **EE** followed by lip shape **U**:*

IA

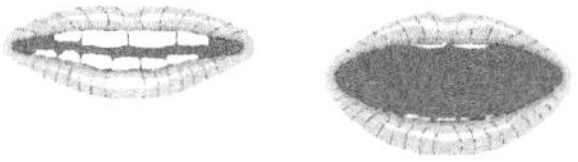

As in: Appeal, Meal, Shield, Associate and Guardian.

***EAR** is formed from lip shape **EE** followed by lip shape **ER**:*

EAR

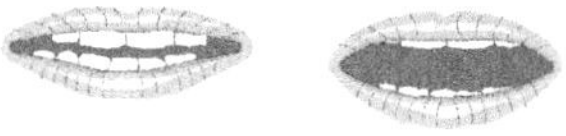

As in: Beer, Fear, Clear, Ear, Dear and Hear.

***EW** is formed from lip shape **EE** followed by lip shape **OO**:*

EW

As in: New, Few, Nude, View, Dew and Avenue.

II *is formed from lip shape* ***A*** *followed by lip shape* ***EE*** *(say AH EE):*

II

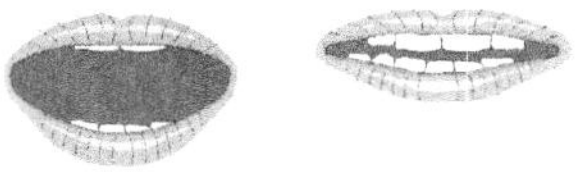

As in: Try, Fly, Buy, Bright, Light and Height.

OH *is formed from lip shape O followed by lip shape OO (say OH OO):*

OH

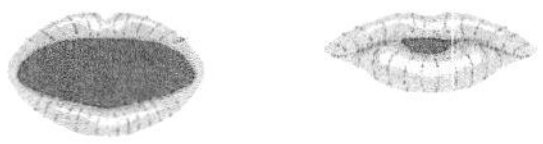

As in: Crow, Show, Motor, Stoat, Loaf and Rope.

OI *is formed from lip shape UU followed by lip shape EE (say AW EE):*

OI

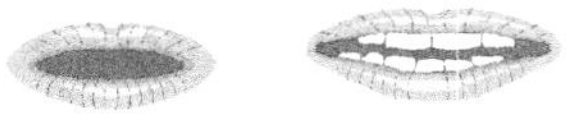

As in: Boy, Coin, Employ, Choice, Boil and Annoy.

URE *is formed when lip shape Y is followed by lip shape UU, followed by lip shape R:*

URE

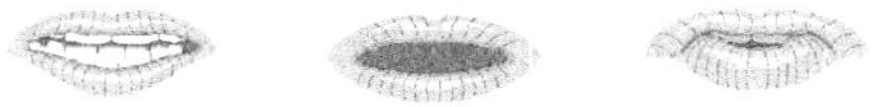

As in: Europe, Culture, During, Cure, Fury and Pure.

Class Practice Phrases:

Bare faced lie	Blame game	Town centre
Take care	Clear vision	New horizons
Try harder	Motor show	Off the boil
Future prospects		

-------------------------------**Activities:**-------------------------------

The clues below are in phonetic text – find their English spelled equivalents in the word puzzle:

CH.ay.n.	P.air.	W.ia.r.ee.	A.v.e.n.ew.	T.r.ii.
SH.oh.w.	CH.oi.s.	K.r.ow.d.	F.ure.ee.	SH.ow.t.
C.l.ia.	N.ew.	URE.oh.p.	C.r.ay.n.	B.r.ay.n.
AY.d.	K.a.r.ia.	CH.ia.		

	A	B	C	D	E	F	G	H
1	E	V	Y	H	O	W	F	R
2	N	A	R	S	H	O	U	I
3	U	E	T	C	S	U	R	A
4	E	C	H	R	O	T	Y	P
5	C	I	O	C	W	D	C	L
6	E	N	A	R	N	R	A	E
7	W	E	N	A	I	A	R	B
8	C	U	E	I	D	C	A	R
9	H	R	O	P	C	E	R	E
10	A	I	N	E	H	E	R	E

Match the words to the correct lip-shape sequences:

Boy, Few, Know, Loud, Pier, Why

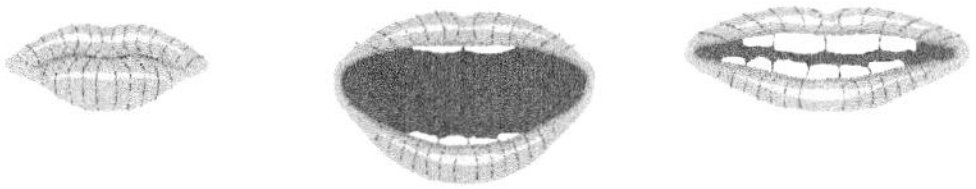

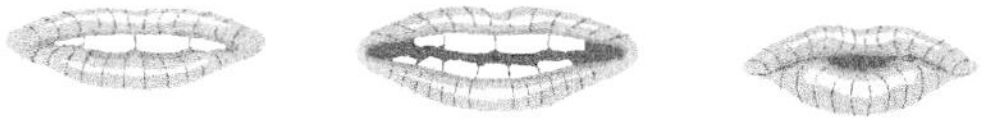

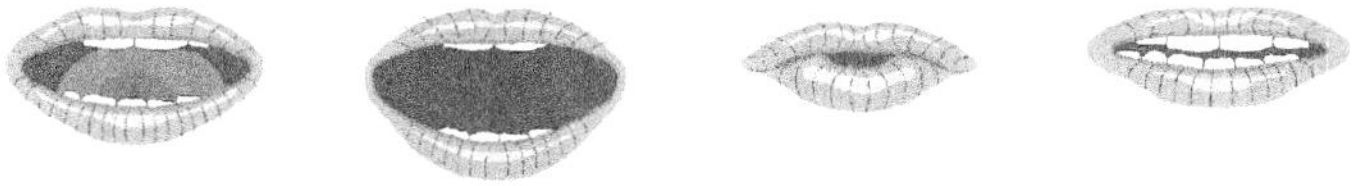

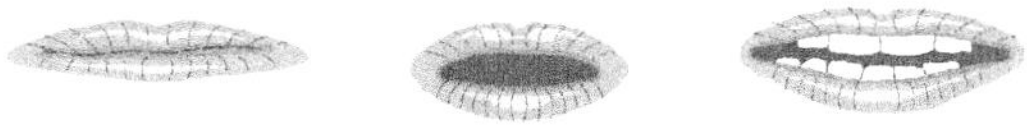

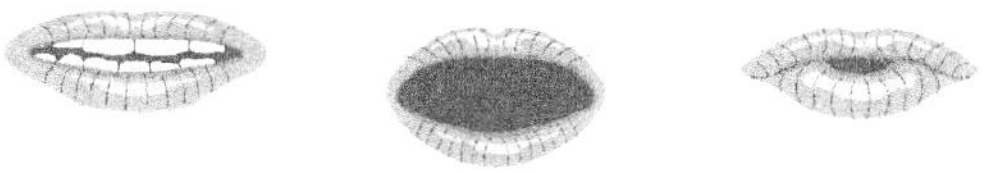

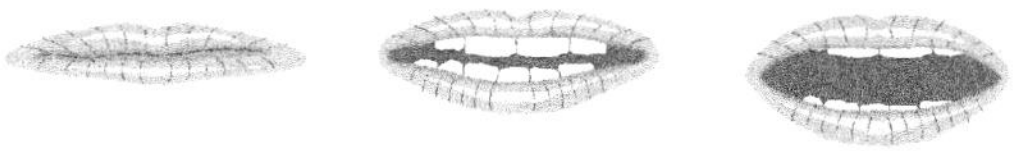

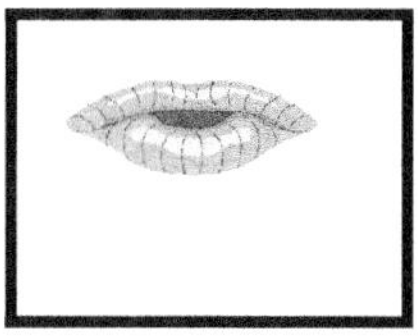

23. Lip Shape OO

accompanies the OO sound and is part of vowels EW, OH and OW

Lip shape OO differs from lip shape W in that with OO the lips push forwards and the aperture is wider.

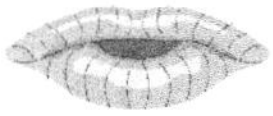

Lip Shape OO

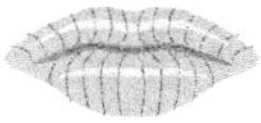

Lip Shape W

The W sound is over in an instant The OO sound is continuous.

OO is rarely used at the start of words.

Observe the following words:

OO in the middle of words

Soup	Troop	Shoot	Tool	Fool
Cool	Pool	Rule	Groove	Smooth

OO at the end of words

Crew	Who	Flew	True	Shoe
Brew	Blue	Sue	Do	Grew

Observe three sliding vowels in the words listed below:

The OO sound is part of the sliding vowel OH as in "grow" – seen on the lips as O.OO:

Loam	Boat	Bloat	Hope	Folk
Show	Know	Flow	Row	Crow

The OO sound is part of the sliding vowel OW as in "cloud" – seen on the lips as A.OO:

Round	Shout	Crowd	Brown	Growl
How	Now	Tower	Loud	Trout

The OO sound is part of the sliding vowel EW as in "few" – seen on the lips as EE.OO:

New	Tune	Dew	Few	Curfew
Newt	News	Stew	View	Pew

Class practice phrases:

A. Too good to be true
B. Stuck in the groove
C. I knew it too
D. Blow me down
E. I doubt that
F. He's browned off
G. Large crowd
H. Like a shoe box
I. Good news
J. It glows in the dark
K. Something to crow about
L. Go down town
M. That's not allowed
N. Nothing to shout about

--------------------------------**Activities:**--------------------------------

Which of the above words is this?

J OO T

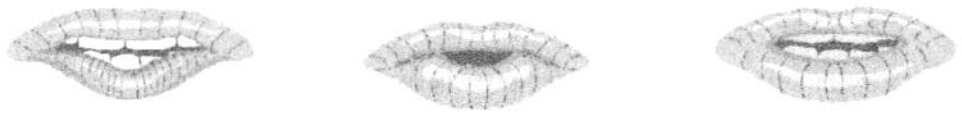

Match the words to the correct lip-shapes

The lip-shape pictures show the first lip-shape seen when the following words are spoken:

Ounce, Over, View, Ewe.

A 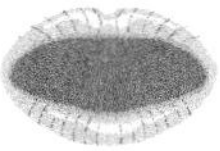 B 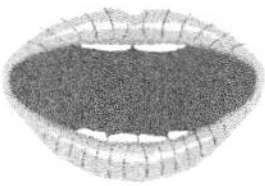 C 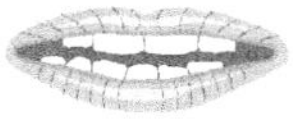 D 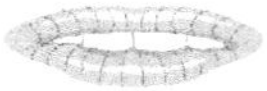

Highlight all the instances of lip shape OO in the following story:

D day anniversary

Bernard Jordan, was a ninety year old veteran of world war two,
He made the headlines last June when he went missing from his nursing home
He was discovered later in France at the D day celebrations.
Sadly, Bernard died back in January.
His medals came up at auction some time later,
They fetched one thousand seven hundred and fifty pounds.
The British buyer of the medals lives in Normandy
He intends to put them on public display in the shop he runs

The clues to the word puzzle are in lip shape text – can you complete the puzzle:

M.l.oh.t.	M.l.oo.	M.r.ow.t.	K.r.ow.t.
K.er.v.ew.	K.r.oo.t	T.ew.	V.ew.
V.oh.k.	K.r.oo.v.	K.r.ow.l.	M.oh.t.
R.ow.t.t.	J.ow.t.	T.ow.er.	T.r.oo.m.
T.r.ow.t.			

	A	B	C	D	E	F	G	H
1	C	B	A	O	L	B	U	T
2	U	R	T	F	E	W	O	D
3	R	O	W	N	D	E	R	N
4	F	W	O	R	C	W	T	U
5	E	D	E	U	L	B	R	O
6	W	G	R	T	O	W	E	R
7	T	R	O	O	V	E	F	T
8	E	O	O	P	K	L	O	A
9	D	U	U	T	G	R	M	O
10	C	R	O	H	S	O	W	L

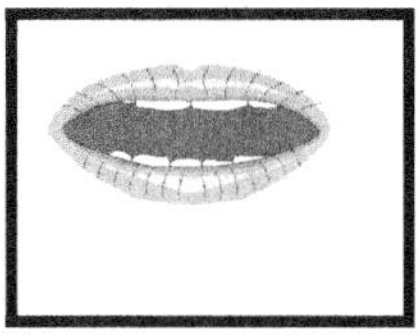

24. Lip shape ER

for ER, AIR and EAR sounds

Lip shape ER frequently occurs in speech. It is the Goldilox lip shape being not too broad and not too narrow. Neither is it wide open as is lip shape A nor is it completely closed up like lip shape M – Lip shape ER is somewhere in the middle of all the extremes. It is the shape that persists on the lips when we pause in conversation to think what to say next.

Observe lip shape ER in these words:

Urchin	Further	Turkey	Bird	Perch
Curly	Turn	Whirl	Church	Early

In speech lip shape ER is often used in words that are written using the letter R. Examples are:

Paper	Better	Perfume	Dirty	Early

In all the words above, lip shape ER is followed by a consonant and this seems to suggest a general rule for predicting the use of lip shape ER and lip shape R.

If the letter R is followed by a consonant lip shape ER is used
If the letter R is followed by a vowel lip shape R is used.

When lip shape ER is preceded by lip shape E it becomes the sliding vowel AIR.

Lip shape E **Lip shape ER**

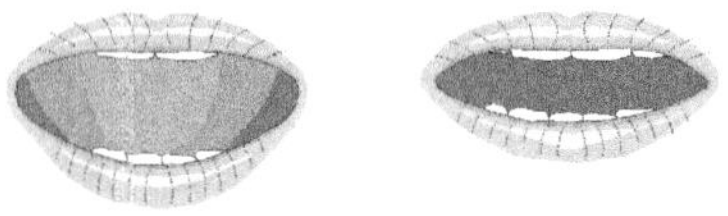

When lip shape ER is preceded by lip shape EE it becomes the sliding vowel EAR.

Lip shape EE **Lip shape ER**

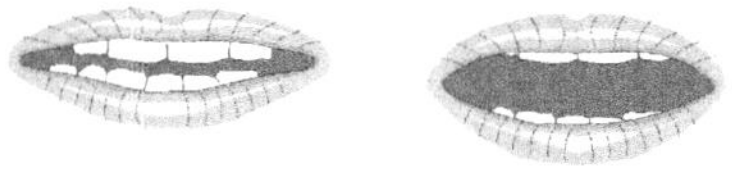

Class practice phrases:

A. Early Bird
B. Stern warning
C. Share and share alike
D. We're nearly there
E. Where there's a will
F. Ne'er do well
G. Upstairs to bed
H. Cold Turkey
I. First come first served
J. Invisible repair
K. Fair shares
L. Happy returns
M. Stand and stare
N. A breath of fresh air

----------------------------------Activities:-----------------------------------

Match the words to the correct lip-shapes

The lip-shape pictures show the first lip-shape seen when the following words are spoken:

Care, Fair, Gear, Journey, Learn, Pair, Urchin, Weir

A 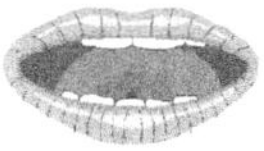 B 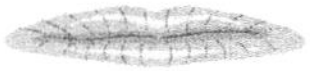 C 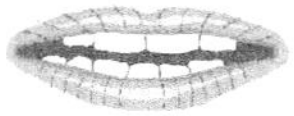 D 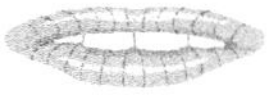

E 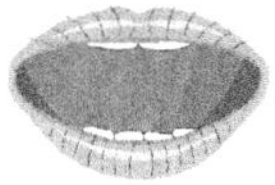 **F** 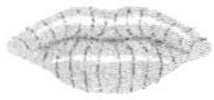 **G** 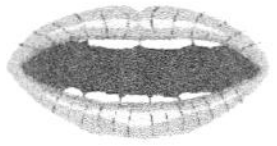 **H** 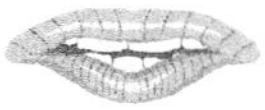

Word Puzzle with words that contain ER or AIR sounds – the clues are in lip shape text:

A.m.j.air.	A.w.air.	K.air.	K.er.l.ee.
ER.l.ee.	V.er.th.er.	M.ay.m.er.	M.er.v.ew.m.
R.e.m.air.	R.e.t.er.t.s.	S.er.v.t.	S.er.v.i.s.
J.air.	S.t.er.t.	U.m.s.t.air.s.	TH.r.e.t.m.air.

	A	B	C	D	E	F	G	H	I	J
1	S	U	P	S	N	R	E	P	A	P
2	R	I	A	T	R	E	H	A	R	E
3	C	U	R	L	S	T	S	A	R	M
4	S	E	R	Y	P	R	I	A	H	C
5	E	S	V	I	E	E	R	A	C	A
6	R	V	E	C	R	F	U	W	E	R
7	R	E	D	E	H	T	M	A	R	T
8	A	P	U	R	R	E	E	F	U	H
9	I	E	T	N	S	A	D	B	E	E
10	R	R	E	A	R	L	Y	A	R	R

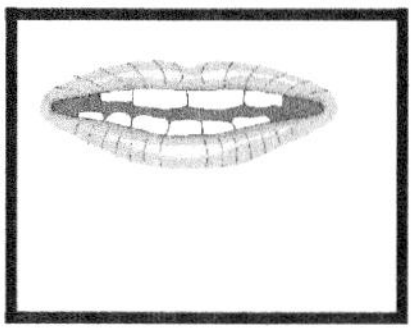

25. Lip Shape EE

accompanies the EE sound and is part of sliding vowels AY, II and OI

Lip shape EE is fairly easy to see. It is wide horizontally and the teeth are clearly seen. It resembles a smile and when a photograph is being taken people are sometimes asked to say "cheese".

Observe the following words being spoken:

Eat	Easy	Eager	Even	Eek
Each	East	Sheet	Treat	Greet
Meat	Neat	Wheat	Lean	Green
Ready	Easy	Agree	Chile	Busy

The EE sound is part of the sliding vowel AY as in "hay" – seen on the lips as E.EE

Observe the sliding vowel AY in the following words:

Hay	Grey	Betray	May	Bay
Tray	Shame	Afraid	Laid	Weigh

The EE sound is part of the sliding vowel II as in "cry" – seen on the lips as A.EE

Observe the sliding vowel II in the following words:

Try	Apply	Fly	Sly	Iron
Hide	Time	Idle	Bridle	Guide

The EE sound is part of the sliding vowel OI as in "boil" – seen on the lips as UU.EE

Observe the sliding vowel OI in the following words:

Toil	Spoil	Boy	Annoy	Joyful
Oil	Soiled	Coin	Join	Employed

Class practice phrases:

A. Eat something sweet for a treat
B. Are you feeling fit?
C. A square meal.
D. Has the mail come yet?
E. How much does it weigh?
F. It is time to try again.
G. Mind how you go.
H. Too many cooks spoil the broth.

--------------------------------**Activities:**---------------------------------

The text below does not make sense. Exchange the words in capitals for look-alike words so that the text makes sense:

Oranges are a delicious fruit containing ANT abundance of vitamin SEA. ONE'S the juicy inner BARN has been eaten IN is usual DO simply discard the outer MEAL. But the MEAL of your orange has SUM uses you MIND not have thought OFF. It has a pleasant citrus fragrance which GAS led to INNS use as ANT air freshener. You simply leave INN lying around IT some inconspicuous PLAYS. Some people have used IN as a body scrub when taking a shower. Others have rubbed INN on their SKIT to deter mosquitoes. Orange skin is edible and HAT be used candied as cake fruit AWE as a delicious STACK. IN can be infused in GOD water to make orange KNEE. The aromatic oils INN contains will infuse into olive oil if left TOO soak for a few days - the oil HAT then be used ASS a salad dressing.

The clues to the word puzzle are all written as sequences of lip shape names – can you complete the puzzle:

	A	B	C	D	E	F	G	H
1	I	O	A	L	J	O	I	N
2	L	Y	P	U	N	A	M	E
3	W	L	P	F	N	T	I	R
4	E	I	O	Y	O	Y	E	E
5	R	R	J	U	C	S	R	A
6	E	W	D	E	S	E	R	C
7	N	E	G	H	H	A	M	E
8	W	E	I	S	T	B	E	T
9	E	D	S	E	E	E	R	R
10	L	I	O	D	I	H	Y	A

U.t.oi.	U.m.l.ii.	M.i.t.r.ay.	K.a.r.ear.
K.ii.t.	J.oi.t.	Ol.l.	J.oi.v.uu.l.
R.e.t.ew.	S.oi.l.t.	J.ay.m.	R.e.s.k.ew.t.
S.t.ear.	T.ii.m.	W.ay.	W.ear.

Highlight the words that contain lip shape EE in the text below:

Fresh-water Eels

There are nineteen species of fresh-water eels in the world. They have long snake-like bodies but although they look like snakes they are in fact fish.

The European fresh-water eel spends part of its life in the sea An eel also spends part of its life in fresh-water streams, rivers and lakes.

Its life begins in the Sargasso Sea where as a juvenile its body is small and transparent

When it has grown large enough to be recognised as an eel but is still transparent it called a glass eel

Glass eels migrate to river estuaries where they experience a mixture of salt water and fresh-water on a regular cycle.

During this time they stop being transparent and take on the colour of and adult eel

Once they have colour they are known as elvers and migrate upstream.

They spend the main part of their lives in fresh-water.

The final episode in the life of an eel is to return to the Sargasso Sea to spawn and give rise to the next generation of fresh-water eels.

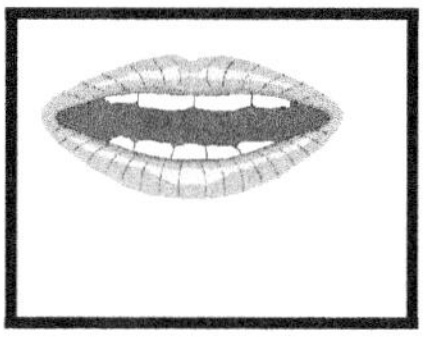

26. Lip Shapes I and II

for the sounds as in trip
and II as in tripe

In lip shape I the width is similar to lip shapes A and EE. The gap between lower and upper lips is midway between A and EE

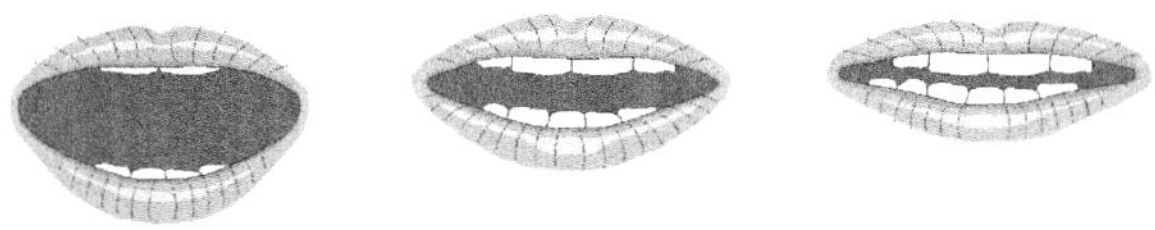
A
I
EE

Observe Lip shape I in the following words:

If	Ink	India	In	Injury	Inform
Fill	Drill	Will	Still	Trill	Shrill

Lip shape I is often used when the spelling is E in words like:

Cricket Carpet Market Crumpet Trumpet

We say "Crickit", "Carpit", "Markit", "Crumpit", "Trumpit"

Don't forget – II is not the same as I

In English spelling we are so used to using the one symbol "i" or "I" to signify I and II sounds and we interchange between them quite automatically.

Now that we are lip reading we have to treat them differently:

The sound I (as in bit) is a single sound and a single lip shape.

Lip Shape I 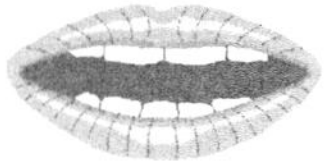 *as in lip, sip or ink*

The sound II (as in bite) is a sliding vowel. It begins with the sound AH and ends with the sound EE.

Try repeating the word "eye" slowly and then speed up – When slow the sound is "AH"-"EE" but when fast it is "II"

The lip reader sees lip shape A and followed by lip shape EE.

Lip shapes II 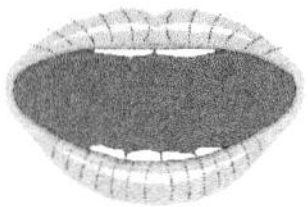 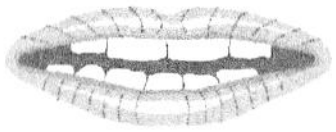 *as in rise or lies*

Observe the lips as the following pairs of words are spoken:

Pill/Pile	Will/While	Slim/Slime	Chilled/Child
Wit/White	Fill/File	Till/Tile	Mill/Mile

Class practice phrases:

A. Biting wind
B. High price
C. In flight service
D. Try it on
E. Thin Ice
F. Mild chill
G. Tight fit
H. Fried fish
I. Fighting fit
J. Chilly wind
K. Bright idea
L. Slight chill

--------------------------------Activities:--------------------------------

Highlight the instances of lip shape II in the following text.

The use of ink for writing began about four thousand five hundred years ago.

The first kind of ink invented was made from lamp black mixed with vegetable oil.

The carbon rich lamp black gave a strong colour that would not fade in the light.

The oil enabled the ink to flow and as it soaked into the writing surface left a sticky deposit enabling the lamp black to adhere.

Indian ink was invented by the Chinese in the fourth century before Christ.

It was made by combining lamp black with ground up charred bones mixed with animal glue.

This was a water based type of ink that could be stored as a solid and mixed with water when it was needed for writing.

It formed a strong bond with the writing surface that does not fade over time.

Match the words to the correct lip-shapes:

The lip-shape pictures show the first lip-shape seen when the following words are spoken:

Earn, Eat, Eye, Imp

A B C D

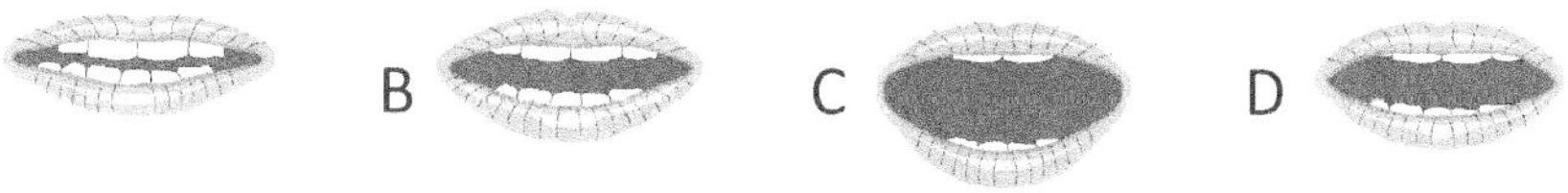

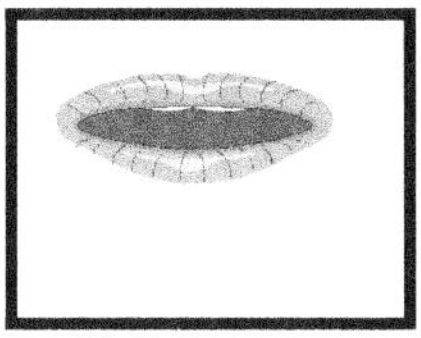

27. Lip Shape NG

accompanies the NG sound

(as in ring, wrong and rung.)

The presence of the NG sound can be detected by the characteristic movement of the lips as they move from shape Nga to shape NGb:

NGa **NGb**

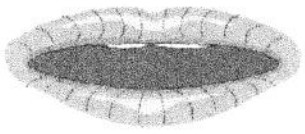 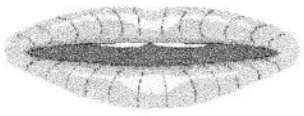

The NG sound comes from the nose and the action takes place deep in the mouth. In many cases the English spelling of NG words contains a vowel followed by "ng".

Observe these words being spoken:

Rang	Ring	Wrong	Rung	Sprung	Wing
Bring	Thing	Fling	Long	Song	Sing

The last sound of these words can be held continuously.

Other NG words are spelled with N followed by K.

Observe these words being spoken

Chink	Link	Tank	Drank	Thank	Ankle
Monkey	Blanket	Anxious	Junk	Extinct	Think

The NG transition is affected by the preceding vowel so it doesn't always look the same.

Compare these pairs of words being spoken:

Ring/Rang Drink/Drank

The transition from lip shape A to lip shape Nga is quite a large movement so is very visible but the transition from lip shape I to lip shape Nga is small as the I and Nga are almost the same. In this case the closing movement is seen as the lower teeth move up to meet the upper teeth.

Class practice phrases:

A. Spring chicken
B. Willing horse
C. Single bed
D. Wrong turning
E. Things to do
F. In the pink
G. To be frank
H. Golf links
I. Soft filling
J. String along
K. Bring to order
L. Lip reading class
M. Sprung a leak

---------------------------------Activities:---------------------------------

Find the listed words in the frame – the word list has been encoded as phonetic text:

	A	*B*	*C*	*D*	*E*	*F*	*G*	*H*	*I*	*J*
1	N	G	E	R	N	K	Y	E	A	N
2	I	L	B	L	A	K	E	L	L	K
3	F	A	E	D	O	N	N	O	E	B
4	G	N	L	E	T	A	G	C	H	L
5	U	N	G	A	N	G	K	N	I	A
6	A	I	M	E	N	R	Y	E	T	N
7	G	H	F	P	K	N	I	F	E	K
8	E	U	U	H	I	B	R	I	G	L
9	G	N	N	T	N	K	K	N	N	E
10	R	Y	G	U	S	E	N	T	A	D

F.i.ng.g.er.	D.o.ng.k.ee.	A.ng.k.l.	TH.i.ng.k.
L.a.ng.g.w.i.j.	A.ng.g.r.ee.	B.r.i.ng.k.	H.u.ng.g.r.ee.
B.l.a.ng.k.	P.e.n.n.ii.f.	M.i.ng.g.l.	E.l.o.ng.g.ay.t.
F.u.ng.g.u.s.	B.l.a.ng.k.i.t.	CH.i.ng.k.	E.n.t.a.ng.g.l.d.

Match the words to the correct lip-shapes:

The lip-shape pictures show the first lip-shape seen when the following words are spoken:
Football, Golf, Hooverball, Lawn bowls, Rugby, Shinty, Stickball, Water polo.

A 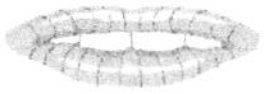 B 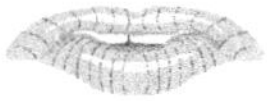 C 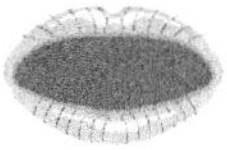 D 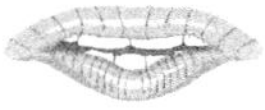

E 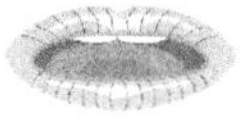 F 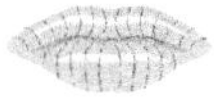 G 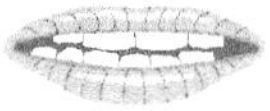 H 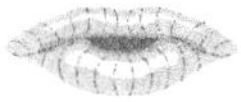

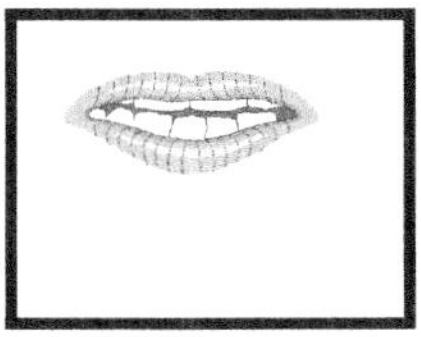

28. Lip Shape URE

accompanies the URE sound

The URE sound is seen as a sliding vowel although the component lip shapes are not all vowels.

Y UU R

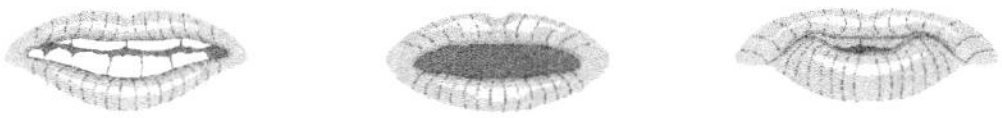

Observe these words being spoken:

During Fixture Cure Luxury Failure Mature
Estuary Lecture Unsure Leisure Injury Fury

Class practice phrases:

A. Buried treasure
B. Insult to injury
C. Life of leisure
D. Endure to the end
E. Future success
F. Miracle cure
G. Manicured nails
H. Amateur team
I. Boring lecture
J. In the picture
K. Natural causes
L. Securely locked
M. Curiosity killed the cat
N. It's a pleasure

-------------------------------**Activities:**-------------------------------

Which of the above words are these?

URE

A L E S Y UU R

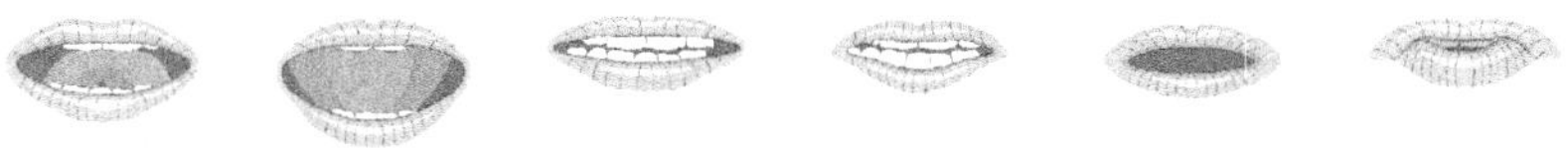

B V Y UU R EE

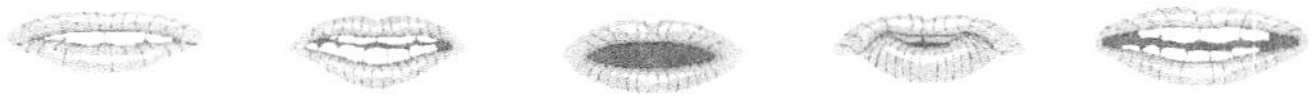

C T

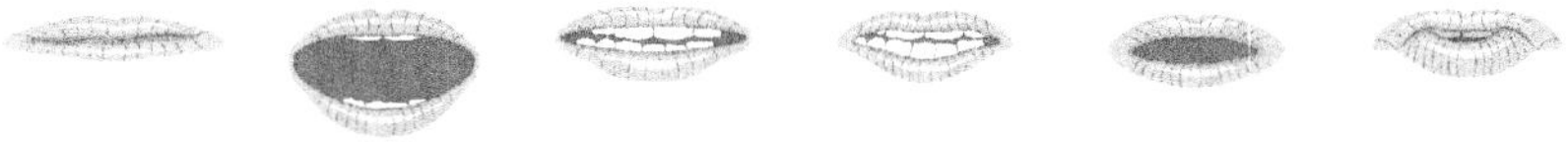

The clues to the word puzzle are all URE words encoded as sequences of lip shape names – can you solve the puzzle?

	A	B	C	D	E	F	G	H	I	J
1	F	C	R	C	U	R	A	C	E	N
2	A	E	E	F	E	I	M	A	Y	T
3	I	R	A	U	R	O	E	T	R	U
4	L	U	T	T	U	S	R	E	U	R
5	E	R	U	Y	C	I	U	T	A	N
6	S	B	O	T	E	T	Y	I	O	N
7	C	U	R	I	N	T	U	R	N	C
8	P	I	E	R	A	D	S	A	A	E
9	O	C	T	U	E	V	S	U	R	E
10	B	S	C	U	R	E	N	T	U	R

A.t.v.e.t.j.ure.
S.e.t.t.ure.ee.u.t.
K.r.ee.t.ure.
V.ay.l.ure.
T.ay.t.ure.
M.i.k.t.ure.
A.j.ure.u.t.s.

A.m.a.t.ure.
S.e.t.t.ure.ee.
K.ure.ee.o.s.i.t.ee.
V.ew.t.ure.
O.m.s.k.ure.
O.m.s.k.ure.i.t.ee.

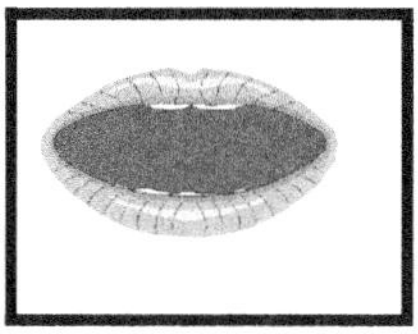

29. Lip Shape U *accompanies U and IA sounds*

Compare lip shape U with other lip shapes:

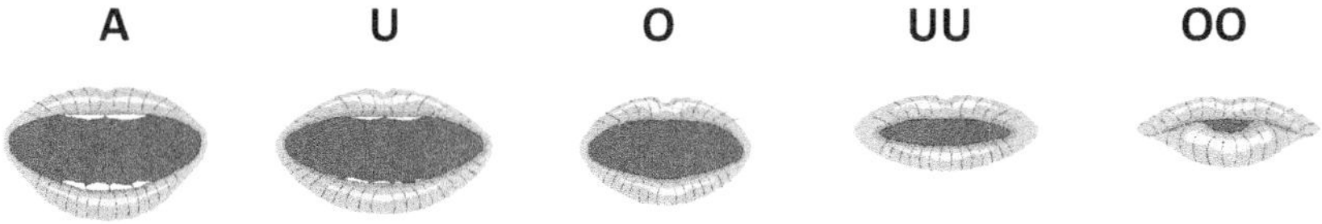
A
U
O
UU
OO

Observe these vowels as the following words are spoken:

Pat Pun Pot Put Boot

Observe lip shape U in the middle of words:

Cup Bump Dull Lust Hump

Observe lip shape U at the start of words:

Upstairs Untrue Above Ugly Affection

Do you think Above and Affection begin with lip shape U?

Class practice phrases:

A. Under the stairs
B. London Underground
C. All above board
D. Cup of coffee
E. Apple crumble
F. Uncomfortable ride
G. Bus pass
H. Upstairs
I. Curry powder
J. Dental Appointment
K. Custard powder
L. Utter rubbish
M. By all appearances
N. Untrue story

--------------------------------**Activities:**--------------------------------

Check if all the following words contain lip shape U:

Love Above Patience Delicious Precious

Which of the above words is this?

A

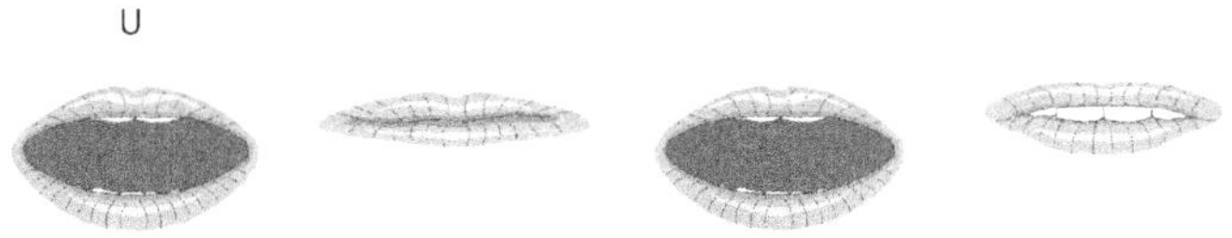
U

When lip shape EE comes in front of lip shape U it becomes the sliding vowel IA:

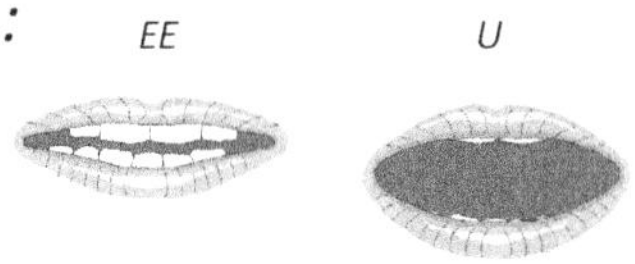
EE
U

Use the mirror to watch the IA sliding vowel as you say the following:

Appeal	Cordial	Hysteria	Idea	Junior
Million	Museum	Real	Really	Zeal

Which of the above words are these?

B

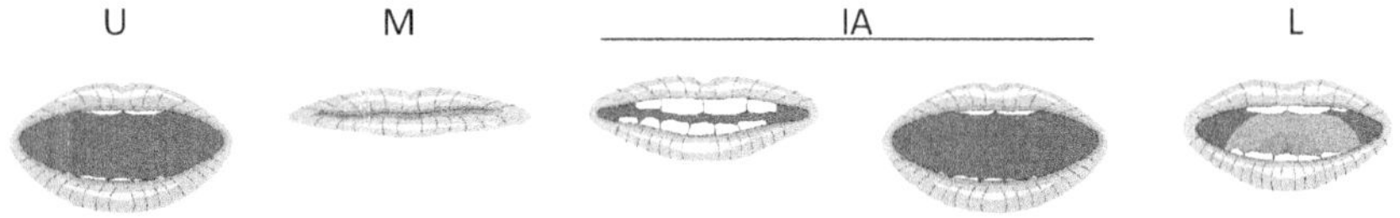
U
M
IA
L

C

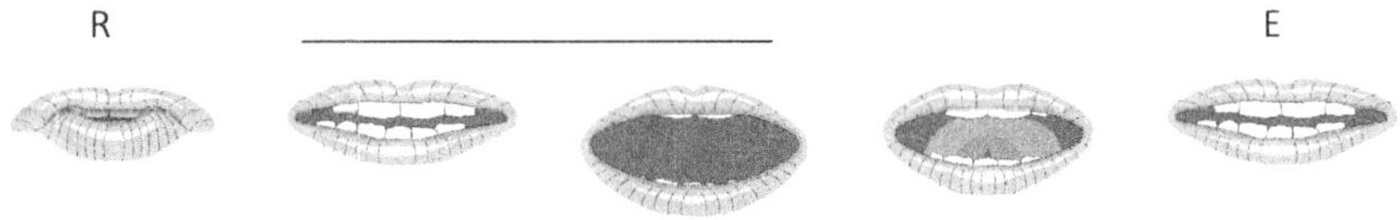
R
E

D

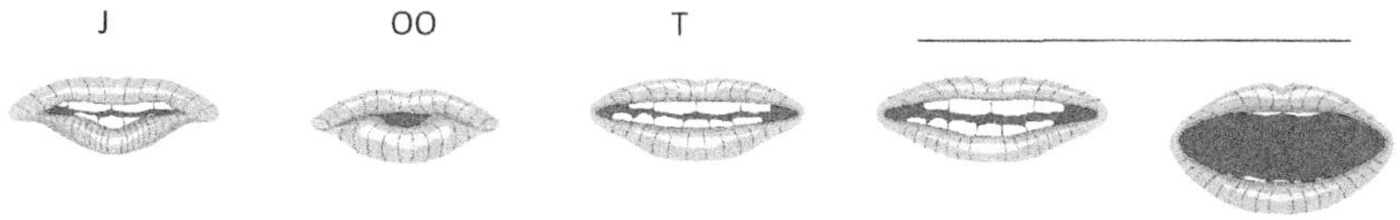
J
OO
T

Highlight all occurrences of lip shape U in the following story:

Mary is fourteen years old.

She was born deaf and has no cochlea in either ear and no auditory nerve either.
The cochlea is a small, snail shaped part of the inner ear that turns sound waves into nerve signals.
These are normally sent on to the brain through the auditory nerve, but Mary has no auditory nerve.
To correct this problem Mary received an auditory brainstem implant.
The implant turns sound into electrical signals which are fed directly into her brain.
Mary can now hear and take part in normal conversation even though she has no cochleas or auditory nerves.
Many deaf people are able to hear again after a cochlear implant operation.
Mary is the first to have an implant that links directly to the brain stem.

Word Puzzle using U words encoded as names of lip-shapes :

K.r.u.m.m.l.	K.u.m.	K.u.r.ee.	T.e.l.i.j.u.s.
S.t.ay.j.u.t.	T.u.v.	L.u.t.t.u.t.	L.u.v.
M.ay.j.u.t.s	M.r.e.j.u.s.	R.u.m.i.j.	T.e.t.t.u.l.
U.t.t.er.	U.t.t.er.k.r.a.oo.t.t.		

	A	B	C	D	E	F	G	H	I	J
1	D	C	P	A	T	I	P	D	E	L
2	O	R	E	C	N	E	R	U	S	I
3	V	U	M	B	L	C	E	O	I	C
4	E	B	U	S	E	I	N	T	A	L
5	U	S	T	A	R	O	E	R	S	H
6	C	C	U	C	D	U	D	U	I	D
7	Y	R	R	U	P	S	L	B	B	N
8	D	E	R	S	L	O	O	N	D	U
9	N	T	A	T	U	V	E	N	O	O
10	U	I	O	N	N	D	E	R	G	R

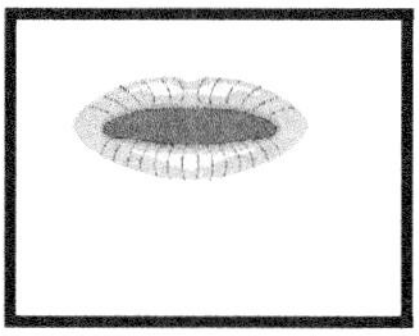

30. Lip shape UU

accompanies UU and AW sounds and is part of the sliding vowel OI

Lip shape UU is midway between U and OO:

U UU OO

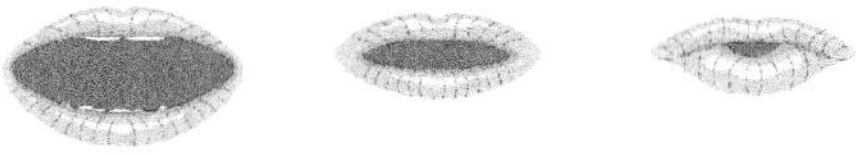

But unlike U and OO it is not recognised in spelling.

Observe these UU words being spoken:

Put	Foot	Butcher	Soot	Good
Should	Could	Pudding	Wood	Look

The same lip shape with invisible internal changes gives the AW sound.

Observe these AW words being spoken:

Awful	Claw	Draw	Floor	Chore
More	Core	Law	Door	Gnaw

Check that these pairs of words have identical lip shapes:

Shorn/Should	Pawn/Put	Warn/Would

The lip shape UU followed by lip shape EE makes the sliding vowel OI.

OI

Notice the action of the lips as in these words:

Choice	Boy	Toil	Boil	Spoil
Toys	Annoy	Joy	Employ	Royal

Class practice phrases:

A. Put your foot in it
B. Little choice
C. More choice
D. Foot in the door
E. Food for thought
F. Claw back
G. Good look
H. Could you come
I. Choice of words
J. Oily rag
K. Good morning
L. Short fuse
M. Good book
N. Calling card

--------------------------------**Activities:**--------------------------------

In the class practice phrases above highlight the words containing the UU lip shape.

Which of the following words do these lip shape sequences represent? ***Awful, boil, boy, pudding, spoil, yourself*****.**

A Y.uu.s.e.l.v.

B UU.v.uu.l.

C M.uu.ee.l.

D

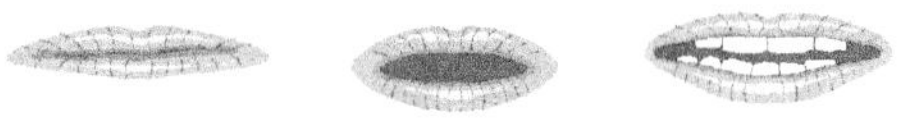

E

S

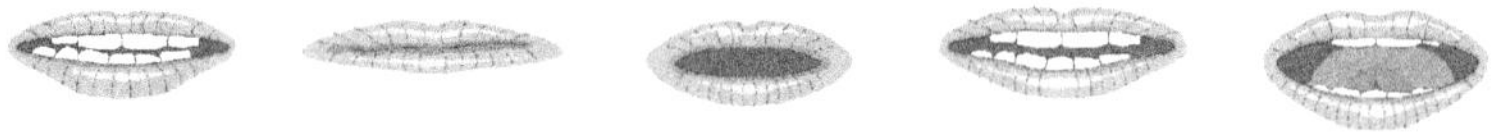

F

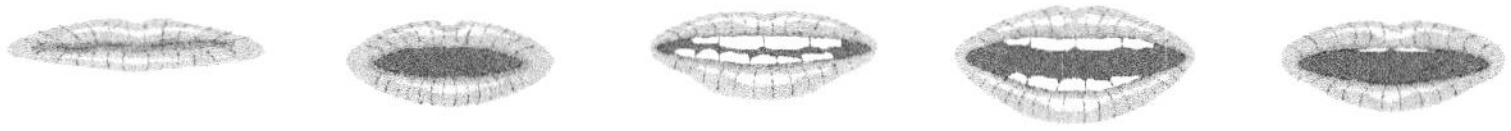
T
I
NG

The clues to the word puzzle are written as a series of lip shapes – can you find all the words?

M.uu.j.er.	K.l.uu.	K.uu.t.	M.uu.
M.uu.t.i.ng.	Y.uu.s.e.l.v.	U.t.uu.ee.	R.uu.ee.y.a.l.
M.uu.ee.	J.uu.ee.s.	T.uu.	L.uu.v.uu.l.
J.uu.t.	S.m.uu.ee.l.		

	A	B	C	D	E	F	G	H
1	F	L	E	L	D	O	I	C
2	Y	O	S	U	C	H	A	E
3	L	U	R	O	H	S	N	N
4	A	U	D	D	S	P	O	O
5	Y	P	C	I	N	G	I	Y
6	O	R	L	G	W	E	L	C
7	B	C	A	N	A	R	O	H
8	U	O	W	M	O	L	O	Y
9	T	U	L	D	R	A	B	L
10	C	H	E	R	E	W	F	U

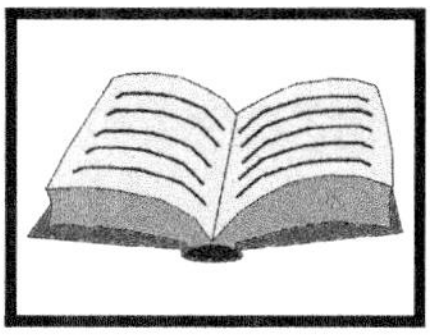

31. Natural Lip Reading

It is often pointed out that most of us, even before we went to any lip reading class, are able to lip read. It seems that we were able to lip read even before we had learned to speak. A researcher named Lewkowicz was studying how babies learn to speak and noticed that between the ages of 4 and 8 months babies look carefully at lip movements and try to copy them. By the age of about 1 year babies seem to no longer need to look at the lips but can manage with hearing only. So it seems that we learned to lip read even before we had learned to speak. And this is a skill we tend to keep in the background and only fall back on it when we find ourselves in noisy situations. Other researchers have noted that deaf people tend to be better at lip reading than those with good hearing. This is not at all surprising because deaf people need, and do, get lots of practice at doing it. When researchers observed how children who are born deaf do at lip reading they found that up to the age of about 14 years children who are deaf are no better at lip reading than children with good hearing. However after the age of 14 the deaf continue to improve their lip reading skills while others no longer show improvement in lip reading skills. But a modicum of lip reading ability remains with most people to be pulled out and used on special occasions like when we try to communicate in noisy places or in situations where talking is not allowed.

One special occasion when the lip reading skill was dusted off and used was noticed by the researcher Harry McGurk at Surrey University in 1976. He was another of those who were interested in how babies come to learn how to speak. Many people working in this field of study find it necessary to look separately at lip movements and speech sounds, and Harry McGurk was looking at a film of someone speaking simple speech sounds while listening to the actual sounds dubbed onto the recording. So the story goes the lips were saying ba ba ba ba ba while the sound track said ba ba ba ba – all very boring and monotonous – but there was a small problem. The technician who had dubbed the sound had made a mistake. Halfway through all the ba ba ba ba sounds he had instead substituted the sounds ga ga ga ga all nicely synchronized with the lip movements on the film. When Harry McGurk and his colleague MacDonald watched the film and listened to the speech sounds they noticed something rather strange. While the lips said ba ba ba ba and the voice said ba ba ba ba all was fine. But when the lips said ba ba ba ba but the voice said ga ga ga ga McGurk actually heard not ba ba ba ba nor ga ga ga ga but instead a third sound – da da da da.

What McGurk had discovered caused quite a stir in the academic world and quite soon almost everyone working in that field of study was repeating the experiment. What McGurk had discovered was that what we think we hear is determined not just by what we actually hear with our ears but is also influenced by what we see the lips doing. When I heard about this research I was struggling to learn to lip read and not getting anywhere. McGurk's work was to me the best news I had heard for a long time. It told me that after all I could lip read – even though I wasn't consciously aware of it, and all that struggling to lip read chunks of text from silent lips in the lip reading class and failing didn't matter. Lip reading silent lips is something very few people have the misfortune to have to do. For most of us hard-of-hearing people, by looking at the lips while listening to the words as best we can, will allow the McGurk effect to take place. We think we are hearing pretty well while in fact the McGurk effect is coming to the rescue to cause the brain to make sense of the disparity between what the ears hear and what the eyes see on the lips – you are lip reading and you don't even notice!

Well that doesn't mean we don't need any more lip reading classes. The McGurk effect is a great help for us hard-of-hearing people – but we do need to hone and practise our skill to make the best of a world of muffled sounds. And don't forget – Watch those lips! If you don't watch the lips the McGurk effect can't happen.

- ***Works with 4-5 month old babies***
- ***Works with speakers of any language***
- ***Works when the audio and video are from people of different genders***
- ***Works when the audio and video aren't precisely synchronized.***
- ***Works better with some sounds than others***
- ***Works less well with vowels***
- ***Works even when the viewer knows what is going to happen***

The McGurk effect –

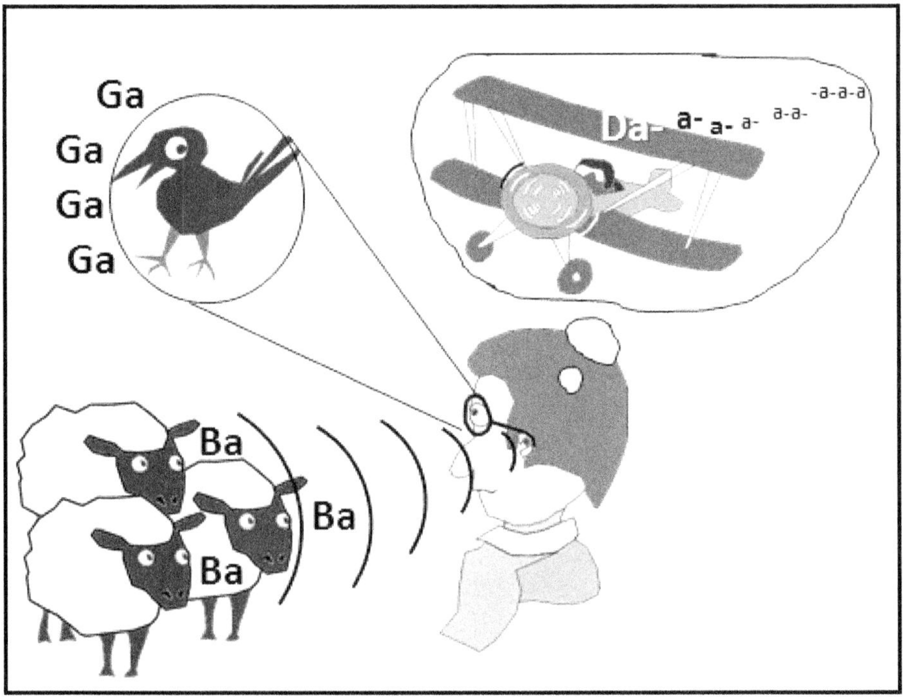
Ga
Ga
Ga
Ga
Da- a- a- a- a-a- -a-a-a
Ba
Ba
Ba

------------------------------Activities:------------------------------

Quiz on the McGurk Effect:

Which statements about the McGurk effect are true – select one or more:

A. The McGurk effect works only with hard-of-hearing people.
B. The McGurk effect does not work with vowel sounds.
C. Works if speaker and listener use different languages.
D. Stops working if sound and vision do not match.
E. Works with children aged 4 to 8 months.
F. Works with teenagers.
G. Can be switched on and off at will.

Look for demonstrations of the McGurk Effect on the internet – Does the effect work if the demonstrator has an accent different from your own?

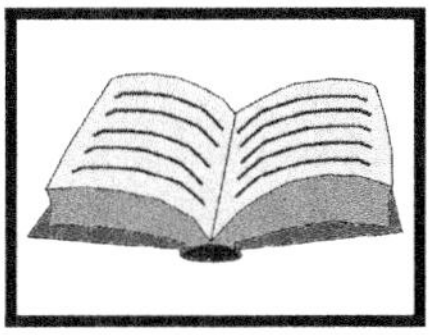

32. Sensing sound direction

I sometimes wish I had eyes in the back of my head like when someone comes up from behind and takes me by surprise. The cyclist overtaking me as I walk along the canal tow-path is an example of this. There I am, day dreaming as I walk along without a care in the world. Then some youngster on a bike comes zooming past and brings me back to the present with a bump. There was one occasion when it was not just me that was day-dreaming. The cyclist was too and there really was a collision.

We have always had a need to be able to sense direction and in particular to know where things and people are in relation to ourselves. In ancient times our ancestors had to hunt to find their food – and if that food was of the kind that could run away it was necessary to know where it was. Even more important was the fact that there were animals that would be interested in hunting you! So being able to see them before they saw you was vital for survival. Well we don't have eyes in the backs of our heads and we can be taken by surprise so our sense of hearing was vital for survival in a dangerous world. But in the present day we don't have many sabre-toothed tigers on the prowl I'm pleased to say. But there are still dangers of a different kind. I am, for instance, very aware of the part my hearing plays as I cross a busy road. To look left and the look right and then to double check takes a lot of head turning and also takes up time so hearing comes to rescue to help us to be aware of dangers our eyes have not yet seen. That car that came round the corner just at the moment I checked in the other direction I can detect with my hearing and yet again I am saved from the danger of a sticky end.

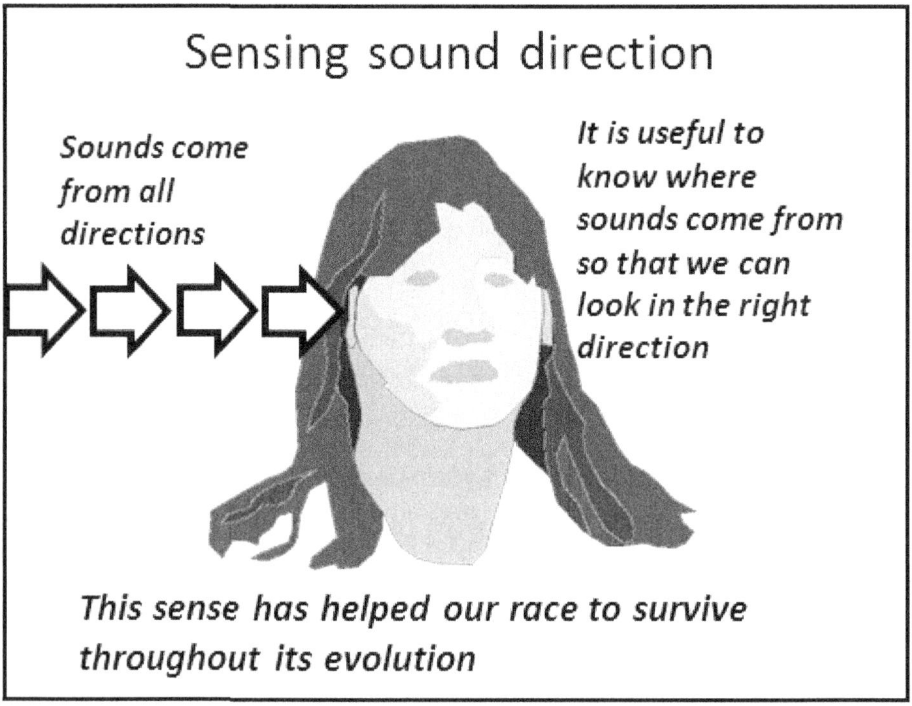
Sensing sound direction
Sounds come from all directions
It is useful to know where sounds come from so that we can look in the right direction
This sense has helped our race to survive throughout its evolution

But how do our ears help us to discern where sounds come from?

Well, one thing we need to remember is that sound travels through the air much slower than light, quite a lot slower in fact. A fifth of a mile a second I was told at school. And compared to light that's pretty slow. Some aeroplanes can go faster than that. But the slowness of sound comes in quite useful in the ears of us even slower humans. We know that sounds come to us from all directions, at a fifth of a mile a second, but the fact that we have two ears – one on the left and one on the right, means that some sounds reach one ear before they reach the other. A sound coming from your left reaches your left ear before it reaches your right ear. And the brain senses the time difference to make you aware that you need to look to the left to see its source.

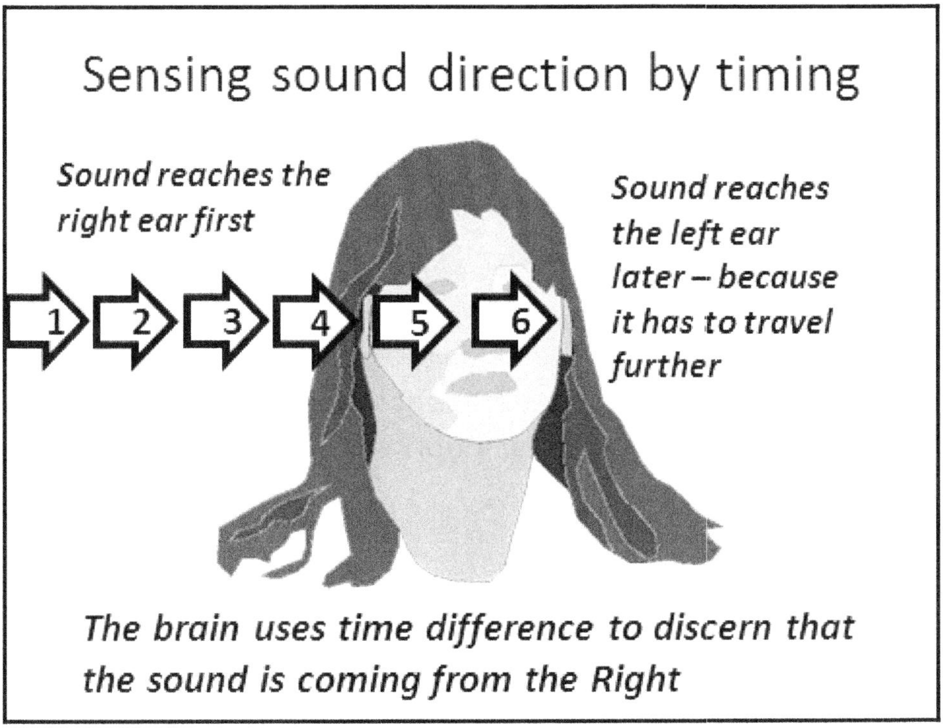
Sensing sound direction by timing
Sound reaches the right ear first
1
2
3
4
5
6
Sound reaches the left ear later – because it has to travel further
The brain uses time difference to discern that the sound is coming from the Right

Our ability to sense where the sound is coming from is down to the fact that we have two ears and that there is some distance between them. A person who is deaf in just one ear is severely disadvantaged in the matter of discerning sound direction. A person with deficient hearing can still discern the direction of the sound of interest provided it can be detected by both ears. And this is done by comparing timings. Another way we discern sound direction uses the fact that sound reaches the ear nearer the source is a little louder than that reaching the more distant ear. Not just because the distance is greater but because the sound, unable to pass through the head has to travel around the head to the ear on the far side. Now sound doesn't like going round corners and when it manages to get to the other side of an object like the head it is much reduced in its loudness. This area the sound has difficulty reaching is sometimes called the head shadow – a bit like the shadows we see on a sunny day but in this case affecting sound instead of light.

You can try the effect of head shadow for yourself by sticking your finger alternately in the right ear and then the left ear and noting the difference in loudness of sounds coming from various directions. The experiment is best done in the open air as indoors the sound can bounce off the walls and confuse the issue.

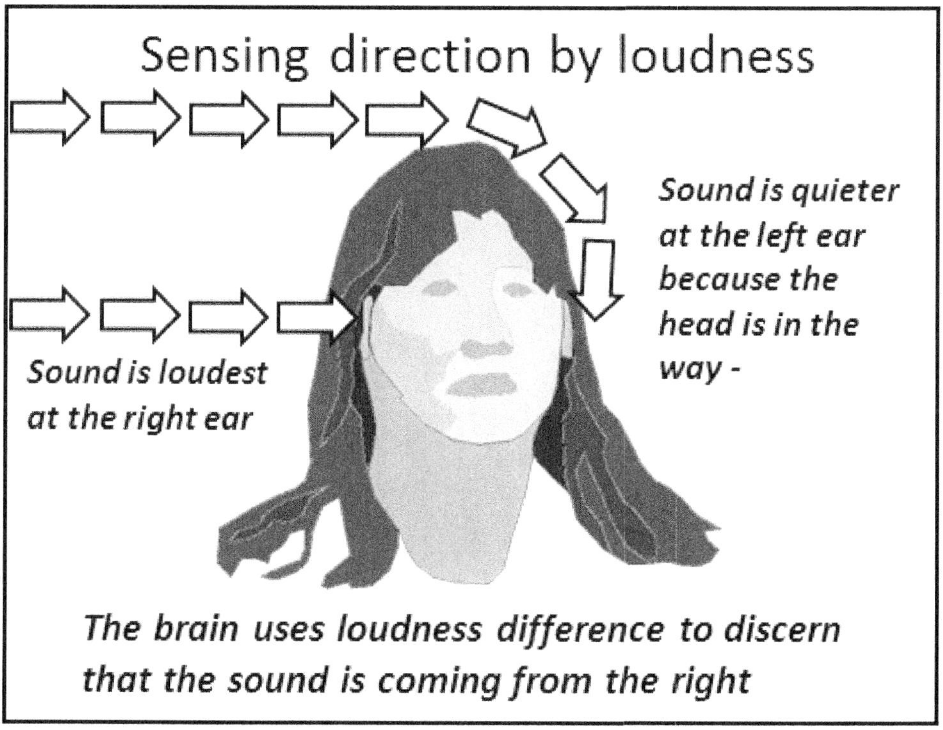
Sensing direction by loudness
Sound is quieter at the left ear because the head is in the way -
Sound is loudest at the right ear
The brain uses loudness difference to discern that the sound is coming from the right

If you did the head shadow experiment you may have noticed that sound heard by the ear furthest from the source was not only quieter but that its quality had changed. In particular you may have noticed that the ear nearest to the sound source heard a full range of notes, both low notes and high notes. But the other ear will have heard the low notes only and the high notes were missing, or reduced. This is because low notes are better at getting around corners than high notes. High notes try to keep going in a straight line. If you are hearing impaired so that you can't hear the high notes at all, the brain is unable to use difference in sound quality to discern direction.

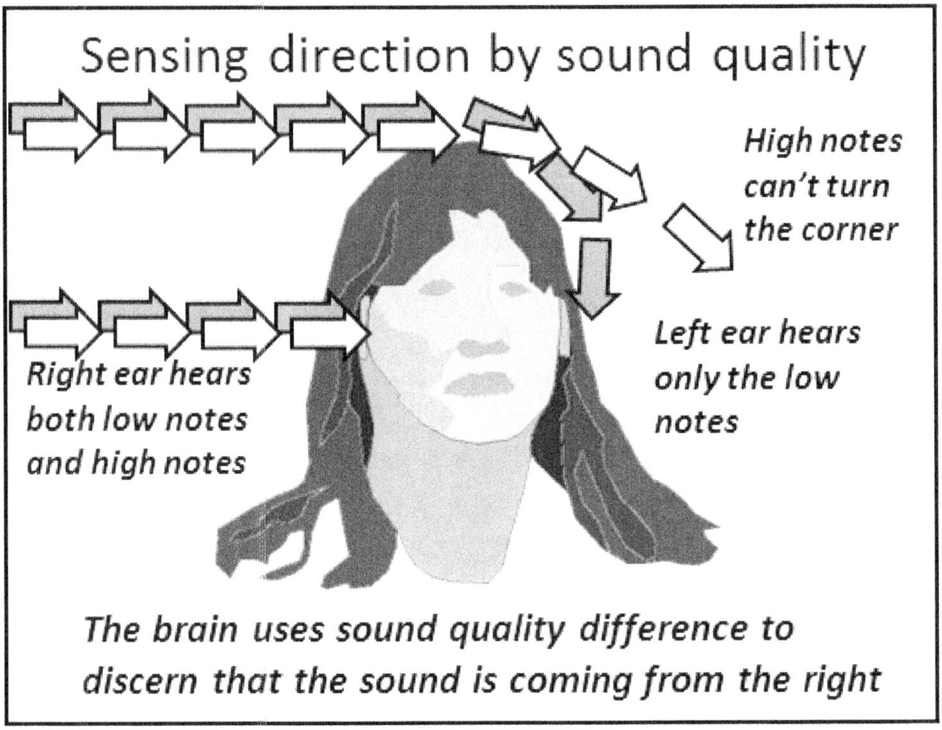
Sensing direction by sound quality
High notes can't turn the corner
Left ear hears only the low notes
Right ear hears both low notes and high notes
The brain uses sound quality difference to discern that the sound is coming from the right

------------------------------Activities:------------------------------

Carry out the head shadow experiment detailed above:

Concerning sounds from the left:

A. Are sounds louder in the left ear than in the right ear?

B. Can you hear high notes better in the left ear than the right ear?

Concerning sounds from in front:

A. Is there a loudness difference between what the left ear hears and what the right ear hears?

B. Is there a difference in the quality of the sound heard by the left ear and the right ear?

When out and about:

Can you discern the direction sounds are coming from better when wearing your hearing aids or not wearing your hearing aids?

Which of these statements is correct? Select one or more.

A. High sounds travel faster than low sounds.
B. Low sounds are better at going round corners than high sounds.
C. Quiet sounds travel slower than loud sounds.
D. Sounds from the left are quieter in the right ear and louder in the left ear.
E. Sounds from the left reach the right ear a fraction later than the left ear receives them.
F. A person who is totally deaf in one ear cannot discern the direction sounds come from.
G. Head shadow is the area sounds cannot reach.

33. Separating the message from the background noise

When most people with normal hearing find themselves in a room with lots of other people all talking to one another, they find themselves able to carry on a conversation with someone nearby in spite of the noisy background - Our ability to do this is known as the cocktail party effect and with this ability we are able to recognise the familiar voice as different from the others and the brain filters out the unwanted voices and pushes them to the background of our consciousness. When we begin to lose our hearing the first thing we are likely to notice is that the cocktail effect no longer works for us and we don't need the audiologist to tell us that we are suffering from cocktail party deafness.
There are several ways the hard of hearing person can seek to minimize the problem of noisy situations and they come under three headings:

1. We can try to visually separate the source of the message from the source or sources of the background noise.

2. We can try to physically separate the source of the message from the source of the noise.

3. We can try to semantically separate the message from the noise.

Visual separation:

It was in 1996 that a researcher named Driver discovered the Ventriloquism effect. He set up a loudspeaker speaking two different stories superimposed on each other using the same actor's voice. With such a jumble of talking it is not surprising that no-one could follow either story.

Driver then set up a screen above the loudspeaker showing the face of the actor telling one of the stories. This time some people managed with some difficulty to follow that story.

Driver then moved the screen to a position well away from the loudspeaker and repeated the experiment. This time a lot more people managed to follow the story and everyone found it a lot easier to do so.

What appears to have happened is that the brain of the listener had been tricked into believing that the voice telling the story was coming from the place the lips could be seen, and as a consequence was able to separate that story out of the jumble of words assaulting the ears.

So next time you find yourself trying to have a conversation in a noisy place try to position yourself so that you can see your companion without a background of other talkers. You will find that the ventriloquism effect helps no end and you can thank Driver for discovering it.

Physical separation:

This trick works better in the open air away from rooms where sound can bounce off the walls. It is about hearing sounds coming from the side and works on the principle that the ear nearest a source of sound hears it better than the ear which is furthest away. This is because the ear is not only closer to the sound but also because the ear on the other side is in what is known as the head shadow. Sound getting to the more distant ear not only has to travel further but it also has to get around the corner before it can get there – and it turns out that low notes are better at doing it than high notes. The brain can also register the fact that the sound reaching the distant ear is not only quieter but that it arrives later – and so can work out which direction it comes from – now try using this idea to work out how best to carry on a conversation as you walk along the street. Do you place your-self furthest from the noisy traffic or let your partner take that position?

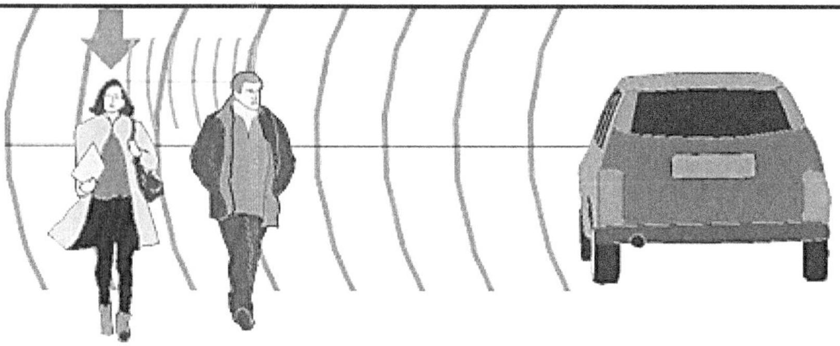

If you place yourself furthest from the traffic:

- ***Your left ear hears both traffic and partner***
- ***Your right ear hears neither very well***
- ***Difficult to separate speech from noise***

Placing yourself furthest from the noisy traffic has its problems:

- Your left ear hears both traffic and partner equally well.
- Your right ear hears neither very well.
- It is difficult to separate the speech from the noise.

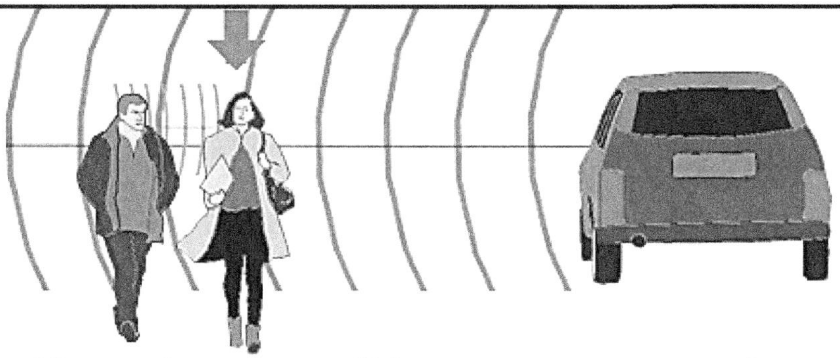

If you place yourself between partner and traffic:

- ***Your left ear hears traffic noise***
- ***Your right ear is shielded from noise by head shadow***
- ***Your right ear hears your partner better***

Better to place yourself between the person you want to hear and the traffic you don't want to hear. That way:

- Your left ear hears the traffic noise but not your partner.

- Your right ear is shielded from the traffic noise because your head is in the way.

- Your right ear hears your partner better as it hears less traffic noise.

Summary

- ***Try to physically separate the noise from the speech you want to hear.***

- ***Position yourself so that the noise is on one side and the speaker on the other – that way the noise is heard better with one ear and the speaker is heard better with the other – the brain will be better able to separate them***

Semantic separation:

Work by Anne Triesman showed that the brain is capable of unconsciously following the meaning of a story. She tried the old trick of bombarding the hearing with two stories at the same time. This time story 1 was heard by the left ear and story 2 was heard by the right ear. Subjects were told to listen to the left ear only and to ignore anything from the right ear.

This worked quite well and subjects were able to follow the one story and ignore the other. All well and good you might think – just concentrate on the ear that hears the message best and ignore the ear where the background noise is loudest – just as we would walking alongside noisy traffic. But here comes the tricky bit – without telling the subjects, in the middle of the stories, the crafty old Triesman swapped over the two stories so that what was heard by the left ear was instead heard by the right and vice-versa. What was quite surprising was that the subjects didn't really notice – they still followed the one story even though it had switched from one ear to the other. Remember they were supposed to be concentrating on what just the left ear heard and ignoring what the right ear heard. Instead they followed the sense of the story from one ear to the other. This is known as semantic separation.

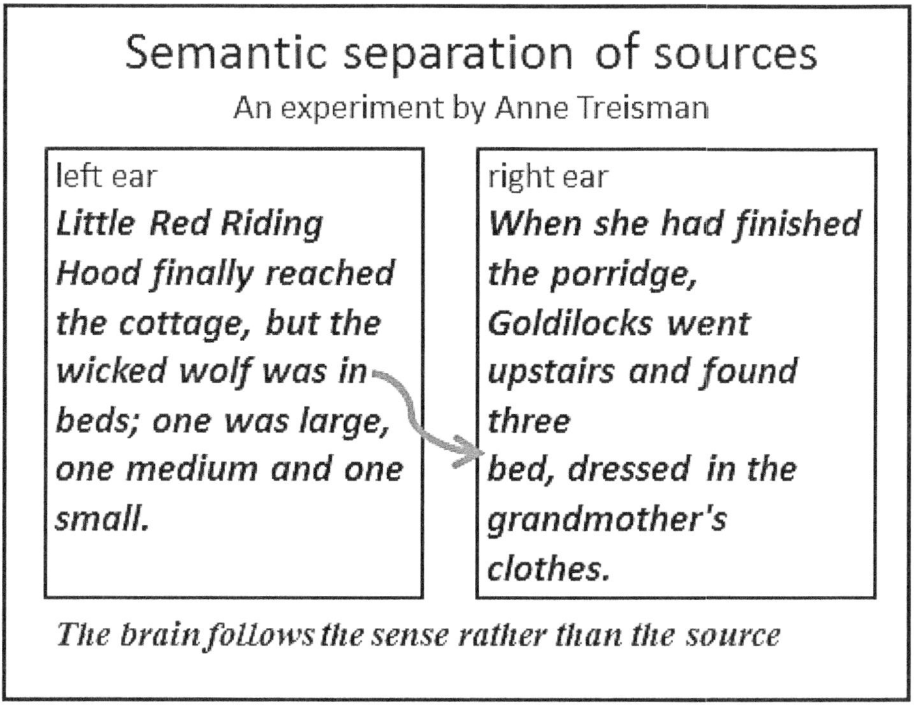
Semantic separation of sources
An experiment by Anne Treisman
left ear
Little Red Riding Hood finally reached the cottage, but the wicked wolf was in beds; one was large, one medium and one small.
right ear
When she had finished the porridge, Goldilocks went upstairs and found three bed, dressed in the grandmother's clothes.
The brain follows the sense rather than the source

Although the ears hear all the sounds the brain is working in the background sorting out the confusion and sending to the conscious mind the stuff that makes the most sense. In order to help the brain do this we should watch the lips of the speaker, (even if we are not lip readers), it will help the brain, working away in the background, to sort out the message from the noise.

Getting the listener's attention .....

- ***Enables them to concentrate on the spoken message***
- ***Gives the opportunity for physical separation***

and once they are looking at the speaker:

- ***Enables semantic separation***
- ***Enables the ventriloquism effect***

The listener does not need to be lip reading

Finally ....

To separate the speech from the noise:

- ***Watch the lips of the speaker***
- ***Even if you are rubbish at lip reading LOOK AT THE LIPS – the brain is better able to separate the speech from the noise, even if the noise is speech.***

--------------------------------Activities:----------------------------------

Try out the traffic noise experiment illustrated on pages 144 and 145:

Does it work for you?

When having a conversation with someone who is facing you try alternately looking at their lips and looking away to see if there is a difference in your ability to hear them.

Fill in the blanks to complete the sentences.

The ability for people to follow one particular voice against background noise is called the C_ _ _ _ _ _l _ _ _ _y effect.

If you can see the lips of the speaker but not see the source of the background noise the V _ _ _ _ _ _ _ _ _ _ _ _ _ _ effect will help you to distinguish the voice of the speaker from the background noise.

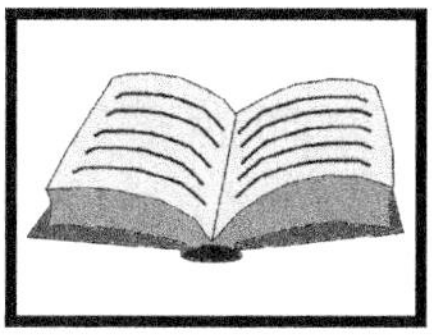

34. How to practise your lip reading skills

Informal practice:

It could be said that we are engaged in practising our lip reading skills every time we engage in conversation, but that is not strictly true. To be engaged in practising it is necessary to be watching the lips of the speaker, not just listening to them. We are not practising our lip reading if we are looking at the eyes of the speaker or looking at their body language. And we are most certainly not practising lip reading if we are looking away at other things. It sounds so obvious but it is true, and we need to keep reminding ourselves to watch the lips.

For myself I have spent many years not staring into people's faces when in conversation – If people stare into my face it makes me feel uncomfortable, so I naturally look away so that I do not have the same effect on them. But now that my hearing is deteriorating I find that I must break the habit of a lifetime and stare back - as discreetly as possible of course. Old habits are difficult to break and I have to keep reminding myself whenever I find I am not hearing correctly.

It's much easier when watching television because people don't stare back at you, but with the television you can't ask the speaker to repeat something. The dialogue just goes on regardless of whether you got the message or not. The television doesn't allow you to engage in the conversation and so there is no feedback to tell you whether you succeeded or failed. But you are practising watching the lips and maybe spotting some of the lip shapes you have been learning about. And if you get into the habit of doing so then there's a good chance the habit will continue when you engage in real conversations – if not, just keep on trying!

Some people try to compensate for their hearing loss by doing most of the talking. But this is not really the answer. If you dominate the conversation you are not engaged in two way conversation you are giving a talk. True conversation involves an exchange of ideas and that requires both communicating your thoughts as well as listening to other people's. Listening and watching the lips is the key to practising your lip reading and you don't need to be chipping in every time.

Engage in active listening by asking for repetition or confirmation:

Would you repeat that please…

Did you say….

Formal practice:

Use a mirror – Whenever you are studying your lip reading have a mirror to hand and get used to using it to check what your lips do as you study the various lip shapes discussed in this book. In some of the lesson notes you are told to use the mirror to check this and that. Use the mirror also whenever you need to clear up a point or can't remember what one of the lip shapes looks like. Mirror work helps to get you familiar with lip shapes and lip movements and that will be a help to you when watching someone else's lips.

With partner or friend – By far the most natural way to practise your lip reading is to engage in conversation with a friend, particularly when your friend is happy to help you by repeating or rephrasing things when asked. You can practise combining what you can hear with what you can see on the lips. It is the best of all worlds because it involves a real exchange of ideas. It is not contrived as in a lip reading class and it doesn't involve the very unnatural process, predominant in all lip reading classes, of speaking without voice. There is opportunity for feedback and in the relaxed situation of a conversation between friends you can engage in active listening without fear of putting someone else to extra trouble.

If your companion is willing to speak without voice to you then you can use the sets of short phrases that are included in most of the lessons for this purpose. In this case keep practising the same set of phrases day after day until you feel you can recognize most of them. Then move on to the next lesson and a new set of phrases.

Lip Reading – I was at a funeral the other day and had managed somehow or other to arrive without my hearing aid. My seat was very close to the front but sheets on the order of service seemed to be in short supply. There were two in my row of seats but both were right down the other end. So in order to follow what was going on I needed to rely on my memory to be able to join in the hymns and I had to listen carefully and watch the speaker's lips to be able hear. I seemed to get on quite well without the hearing aids and understood what was going on. Then a lady with a rather quiet voice came to the front to speak. I still heard her voice and understood the message until the point when her hand obscured her mouth. Then although I still heard her voice, I could understand nothing.

This is a demonstration of how lip reading can help us in everyday life and also a demonstration of how easily its advantages can be lost if for whatever reason we do not see the lips of the speaker.

You can check and practise your ability to lip read by getting a partner to read to you using their normal voice. You, as the lip reader, should watch their lips as they read. With your hearing aids in use reduce the volume bit by bit until you can no longer understand what is being read. Then push the hearing aid volume up until you just begin to understand.

As you carry on listening and watching the lips you are engaged in lip reading. To check that this is so look away from the lips but still listen. If you have been lip reading you will still hear the voice but be unable to understand the message. Looking back at the lips again your understanding of the message should be restored.

If this works for you then doing it frequently should improve your lip reading.

1. ***Listen and watch the lips.***
2. ***Turn down hearing aid volume until you can no longer understand what is being read.***
3. ***Turn hearing aid volume up until you can just understand.***
4. ***Check:***

   Look away and you will no longer understand.

   Look again and your understanding will be restored

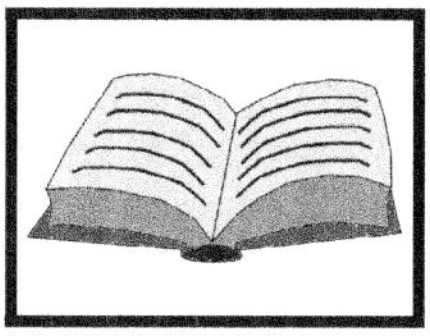

35. Reading silent lips

Many people who have attended lip reading classes will have been faced with the situation where the lip reading teacher speaks without voice while the students try to understand what the silent lips are saying. This is a most unnatural situation and one in which (unless you are profoundly deaf), you are unlikely to encounter in everyday life. For most of us hard of hearing people our lot is to hear some of the speech and lip read what we can't hear. Interpreting what silent lips are saying is quite difficult for anything more than short sentences or phrases spoken in context. But, because there is no viable alternative, most lip reading students have to endure silent lips in their lip reading classes.

It seems to me that a lot of students feel they are failing to learn when they fail to lip read silent lips – and are particularly put off when someone else in the class shouts out the answer before they even have a chance at a second attempt. So it's important to recognize that ability to lip read is not measured by how well you do at reading silent lips but by how well you do when using your residual hearing and interpreting not quite so silent lips. The moral seems to be don't be put off by the problems of silent lips – they seem to be a part of lip reading classes we can't escape from.

On a happier note modern techniques for revealing where and when different parts of the brain become active have recently provided a window on the process of lip reading. One example is functional magnetic resonance imaging (fMRI). This technique has revealed that areas of the brain that respond to hearing speech are also activated in a person viewing lips making speech movements *in the absence of sound*. Such findings reveal that although some parts of the brain are associated with speech and other parts with vision, there are connections between them so that speaking without voice can, and does, activate those connections.

> ***The part of the brain that responds to speech is also activated in a person viewing moving lips.***

Chapter 1 Answers

Lip shapes and Sounds:

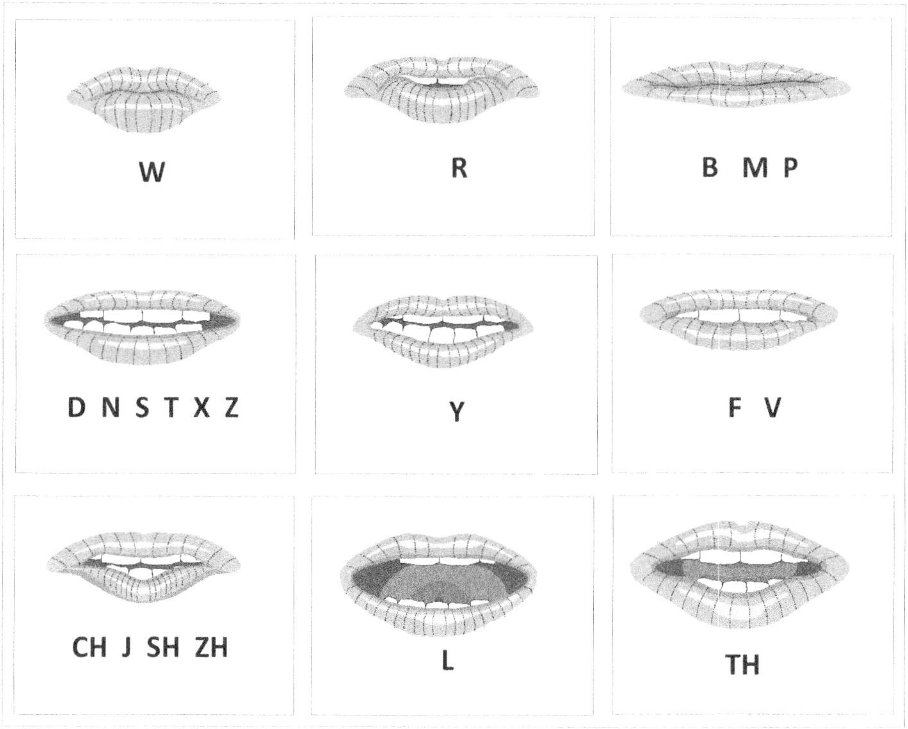
W
R
B M P
D N S T X Z
Y
F V
CH J SH ZH
L
TH

Chapter 2 Answers

Phonetic words:

N.ay.m.	=	Name	K.o.p.ee.	=	Copy
N.e.x.t.	=	Next	B.i.g.	=	Big
S.m.aw.l.	=	Small	T.ii.n.ee.	=	Tiny
L.ah.s.t.	=	Last	L.ah.f.	=	Laugh
T.ii.d.ee.	=	Tidy	G.ay.t.	=	Gate
H.aw.s.	=	Horse	F.ee.l.d.	=	Field

Solution to word puzzle:

	A	B	C	D	E	F	G	H	I	J
1	**C**	E	T	L	I	N	**T**	R	E	E
2	O	D	S	A	**C**	G	R	E	**A**	E
3	**W**	R	E	R	T	**S**	U	**S**	R	R
4	**L**	T	E	P	A	**F**	T	A	O	O
5	I	K	E	P	T	I	X	I	L	P
6	**C**	R	I	S	I	Y	R	**T**	E	L
7	N	O	**P**	O	O	N	O	O	N	A
8	**T**	O	T	N	R	A	T	**M**	O	W
9	A	**L**	A	B	O	A	I	N	**H**	E
10	I	L	O	R	**T**	R	T	N	U	R

T.r.ee. = G1-Tree
C.oh.d. = A1-Code
L.ii.k. = A4-Like
T.ay.l.er. = A8-Taylor
M.oh.er. = H8-Mower
S.ay.l.er. = H3-Sailor
S.t.ay.sh.u.n.= F3-Station
R.e.s.l.i.ng. = A3-Wrestling
C.ah.p.e.t. = E2-Carpet
C.r.i.s.p. = A6-Crisp
P.o.n.t.oo.n. = C7-Pontoon
L.a.b.o.r.a.t.aw.r.ee.
= B9-Laboratory
F.i.x.t.ure. = F4-Fixture
AIR.u.p.l.ay.n.= I2-Aeroplane
T.oo. = H6-To
T.r.ay.n. = E10-Train
H.u.n.t. = I9-Hunt

Chapter 3 Answers

Matching the words on the list to the correct lip-shapes?

1 Wednesday 2 Saturday 3 January 4 October

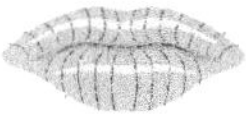 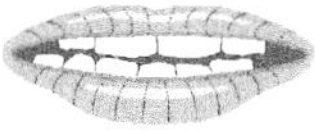 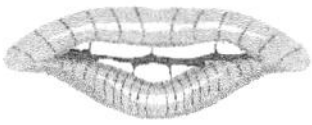 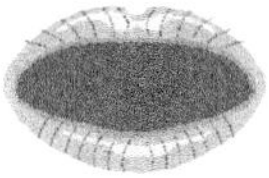

5 Monday 6 Year 7 Friday 8 Thursday

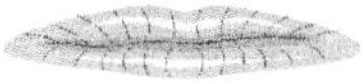 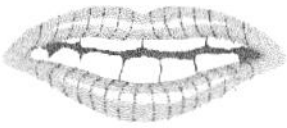 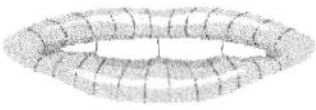 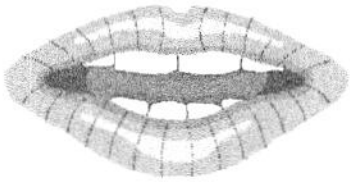

Chapter 4 Answers

Matching the words on the list to the correct lip-shapes?

1 Rabbit 2 Walrus 3 Bulldog 4 Lovebird

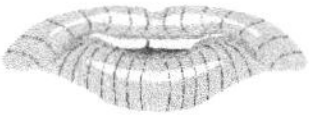 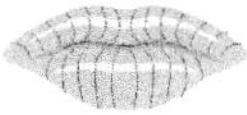 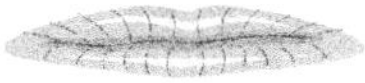 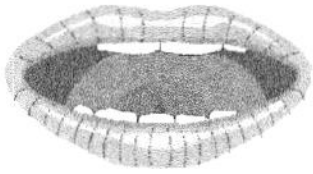

5 Yak 6 Chicken 7 Donkey 8 Frog

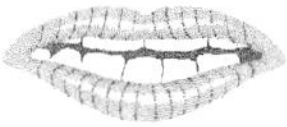 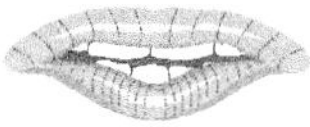 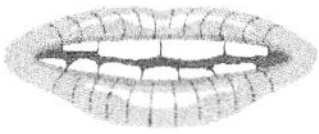 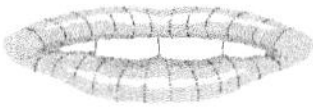

Chapter 5 Answers

Matching the words on the list to the correct lip-shapes

1 Ugly   2 Extra   3 Urban   4 Apple

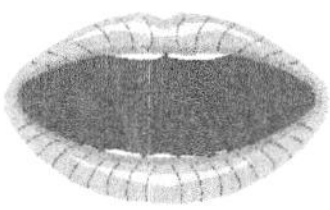
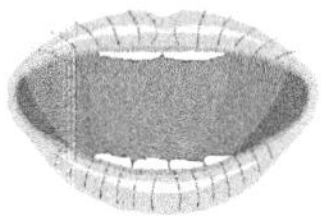
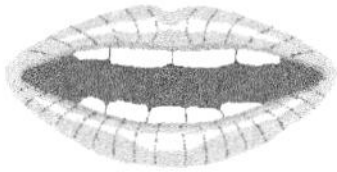
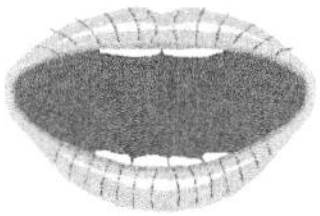

5 Order   6 India   7 Orange   8 Easy

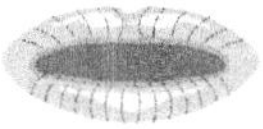
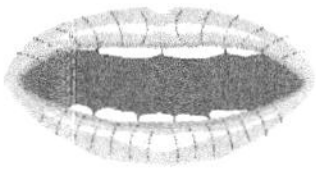
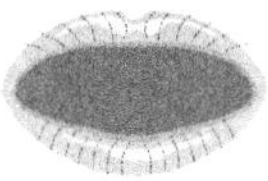
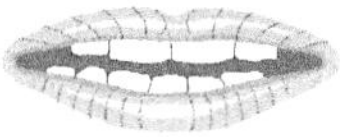

Chapter 6 Answers

Highlighting:

The **toy** **fair** will be held this year at the **leisure** centre on **April** fifteenth. Exhibitors are asked to set up **their** stalls between seven and **nine** in the morning. The public will be admitted at **nine** o'clock. The **fair** **closes** at six pm.

Toy	*contains sliding vowel*	*OI*
Fair	*contains sliding vowel*	*AIR*
Leisure	*contains sliding vowel*	*URE*
April	*contains sliding vowel*	*AY*
Their	*contains sliding vowel*	*AIR*
Nine	*contains sliding vowel*	*II*
Closes	*contains sliding vowel*	*OH*

Word Puzzle

	A	B	C	D	E	F	G	H	I	J
1	**F**	R	A	Y	S	U	**M**	**S**	H	**D**
2	**F**	L	**E**	C	I	**F**	E	R	A	E
3	**H**	Y	M	P	**B**	R	O	W	**S**	W
4	E	A	R	L	E	I	R	N	H	**C**
5	**S**	**V**	Y	O	E	A	T	U	O	H
6	H	O	I	C	R	P	E	N	I	A
7	O	W	**C**	E	**N**	E	**R**	**R**	**G**	O
8	E	R	U	R	E	U	R	E	**D**	U
9	H	E	G	H	**D**	R	O	A	R	R
10	**W**	**H**	I	N	I	A	N	G	N	I

B.ear.	= E3-Beer	H.ear.	= A3-Here
CH.ay.n.	= J4-Chain	H.ii.	= B10-High
C.ure.	= C7-Cure	M.ew.z.i.k.	= G1-Music
D.ew.	= J1-Dew	N.ure.o.n.	= E7-Neuron
D.r.ay.n.	= E9-Drain	R.ear.	= H7-Rear
D.ure.i.ng.	= I8-During	R.e.p.air.	= G7-Repair
E.m.p.l.oi.	= C2-Employ	SH.air.	= H1-Share
F.l.ii.	= A2-Fly	SH.ow.t.	= I3-Shout
F.r.ay.	= A1-Fray	SH.oh.w.	= A5-Show
F.r.ow.n.	= F2-Frown	V.oi.s.	= B5-Voice
G.oh.	= I7-Go	W.air.	= A10-Where

Chapter 7 Answers

Words that look similar:

Make/Bake
Pike/Bike/Mike
Praise/Braise
Memory/Peppery
Pail/Mail/Bail
Boast/Most/Post

Note also:

Match/Patch/Badge *(CH and J also look the same)*
Beat/Meet/Bean/Peat/Mean *(T and N also look the same)*

Interpretations that make sense:

Beauty parlour
Bread pudding
He wore a club badge on his lapel.
She filled the big pan with water.
Camping holiday
He went to school by bike.
Please post my letters for me.
Pass the Parcel
Shepherd's pie

Chapter 8 Answers

Identity of lip shape sequences:

A = Brief B= Cover C = Tough D = Village

Highlight text on the feverfew plant

Unvoiced = underlined italic
Voiced = **underlined bold.**

The *f*e**v**er*f*ew plant is a member o**f** the daisy *f*amily.
It is widely distributed throughout Europe North America and Australia.
*F*e**v**er*f*ew is a perennial plant that *f*lowers *f*rom July to October in the Northern hemis*ph*ere.

In ancient times *f*e**v**er*f*ew was used to treat *f*e**v**ers but experiments in more recent time ha**v**e not *f*ound it to be e*ff*ecti**v**e. Nowadays *f*e**v**er*f*ew is belie**v**ed to help pre**v**ent migraines and se**v**eral studies suggest that it is e*ff*ecti**v**e *f*or that purpose.

The treatment tried out by migraine su*ff*erers was to eat two or three *f*resh lea**v**es daily.

Alternati**v**ely *f*e**v**er*f*ew supplements can be obtained *f*rom health *f*ood shops.

Word puzzle:

	A	B	C	D	E	F	G	H	I	J
1	P	A	R	G	**F**	R	A	**C**	S	E
2	H	**F**	E	O	I	A	H	R	A	E
3	H	C	T	T	S	V	**P**	T	U	R
4	**F**	**P**	H	O	H	A	N	U	O	**R**
5	A	**V**	F	R	**C**	U	R	**F**	U	G
6	C	A	**V**	O	W	N	F	E	W	H
7	E	L	A	**F**	A	S	H	I	O	N
8	E	U	S	**R**	**S**	T	U	**T**	O	U
9	I	**V**	E	E	F	U	F	F	H	G
10	L	L	A	G	E	G	E	I	N	G

C.er.f.ew. = E5-Curfew
R.e.f.ew.j. = D8-Refuge
R.u.f. = J4-Rough
S.t.u.f.i.ng. = E8-Stuffing
T.u.f. = H8-Tough
V.a.l.ew. = B5-Value
V.ah.z. = C6-Vase
V.i.l.i.j. = B9-Village
F.oh.t.u.g.r.ah.f. = B4-Photograph

F.ay.s. = A4-Face
F.a.sh.u.n. = D6-Fashion
F.e.ch. = B2-Fetch
F.i.sh. = E1-Fish
F.r.ow.n. = C5- Frown
F.ew.t.ure. = H5-Future
F.r.ay.z. = G3-Phrase
C.a.r.u.v.a.n. = H1-Caravan

Chapter 9 Answers

Mirror exercise:

The words that use lip shape W are in bold type, the others use lip shape OO.

Twine	Newt	Lower	Shower	**Swift**
Swan	Crowd	**Dwelling**	Snowing	Newest

Lip shape pictures:

A = WORTH B =LOWER C = MOW D = SWELL

Highlighting:

Underline = *Lip shape W*

Underline/bold = *lip shape OO used instead of lip shape W.*

Underline/italic = *Words spelled with O but spoken with lip shape W.*

A wolf was on the loose near the Zoo after breaking through a wire fence and vanishing into the woods.
Police cordoned off a wide area of undergro**w**th while they searched for the missing wolf.

The alarm was raised when five wolves escaped through a damaged fence while a sixth wolf stayed behind.
All but one were accounted for but t**wo** had to be shot dead.
One of the wolves returned of its o**w**n accord another was recaptured.
The remaining wolf was thought to be sheltering in the nearby woods.

Word puzzle :

	A	B	C	D	E	F	G	H	I	J
1	T	E	D	E	I	C	**S**	**F**	L	O
2	S	A	**W**	W	U	K	W	A	L	W
3	I	N	R	O	**Q**	L	S	H	L	E
4	W	G	R	O	**B**	Y	I	W	O	R
5	O	E	Z	E	R	S	**W**	**Q**	U	O
6	**T**	E	**W**	I	N	T	E	R	E	T
7	**D**	W	**T**	I	N	G	E	H	I	W
8	W	E	L	L	N	K	L	T	N	O
9	U	E	A	W	I	**W**	O	R	G	L
10	Q	**S**	K	**T**	**N**	O	W	**B**	E	L

Q.oh.t.	= H5-Quote	W.i.sh.	= G5- Wish
W.ay.s.t.	= C2-Waste	W.i.n.t.er.	= C6-Winter
Q.i.k.l.ee.	= E3-Quickly	W.er.th.	= F9-Worth
S.q.ee.k.	= B10-Squeak	S.w.o.l.oh.	= G1-Swallow
T.w.i.n.k.l.	= D10-Twinkle	T.w.ee.z.er.z.=	C7-Tweezers

D.w.e.l.i.ng. = A7-Dwelling B.e.l.oh.i.ng.= H10-Bellowing
F.l.ow.er. = H1-Flower B.o.r.oh.d. = E4-Borrowed
T.ow. ....= E10-Now

Chapter 10 Answers

Matching words in normal and lip shape form:

Barter = M.ah.t.er. Butter = M.u.t.er.
Frequent = V.r.ee.w.n.t. Harbour = K.ah.m.er.
Master = M.ah.s.t.er. Parlour = M.ah.l.er.
Pastry = M.ay.s.t.r.ee. Prudent = M.r.ew.t.u.n.t.
Puddle = M.u.t.l. Putty = M.u.t.ee.
Quibbling = W.i.m.l.i.ng. Simple = S.i.m.m.l.
Wafer = W.ay.v.er. Wager = W.ay.j.er.
Willing = W.i.l.i.ng.

Word puzzle:

	A	B	C	D	E	F	G	H	I	J
1	S	R	U	O	V	**C**	M	B	L	E
2	D	D	I	L	A	R	U	K	N	I
3	U	G	N	**F**	**P**	O	C	E	M	R
4	**P**	L	U	**H**	O	L	I	N	A	**D**
5	**P**	G	F	E	P	**P**	L	I	D	A
6	U	N	I	D	D	E	O	**H**	T	Y
7	R	P	L	E	E	R	F	E	C	G
8	**C**	I	N	D	**W**	L	O	P	I	N
9	H	W	**L**	I	G	**S**	P	S	A	**W**
10	O	I	C	E	H	T	**L**	O	S	T

M.l.ee.s.m.uu.t = E3-Policeman J.oi.s. = A8-Choice
M.uu.t.i.ng.= A4-Pudding K.o.l.i.t.ay. = H6-Holiday

W.o.s.m. = J9-Wasp	S.l.oh.m.i.ng. = F9-Sloping
M.er.v.e.k.t. = F5-Perfect	K.oh.m.v.uu.l.=D3-Hopeful
K.r.u.m.m.l. = F1-Crumble	T.r.i.ng.k. = J4-Drink
L.ii.t. = C9-Light	V.l.ay.v.er.s . = D3-Flavours
L.o.s.t. = G10-Lost	W.e.t.i.ng. = E8-Wedding
M.er.m.l. ...= A5-Purple	W.i.n.t. = B9-Wind

Chapter 11 Answers

Matching names to lip shapes:

A – William	B = Larry	C = Paul	D = Oliver
E = Sylvia	F = Rachael	G = Jill	H = Felicity

Lip shape text:

A = A level playing field
B = University Challenge
C = Lip reading is difficult if people shout
D = Lip reading is possible only when people face you

Chapter 12 Answers

Matching words to lip shapes

The lip-shape pictures show the first lip-shape seen when the following words are spoken:

WAX LAND APPLE FAST

A 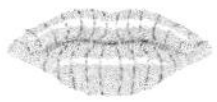 B 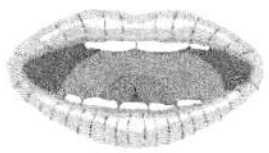 C 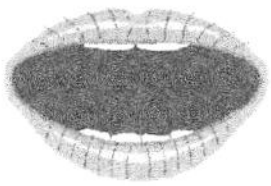 D 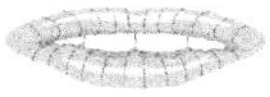

TRAMP

E 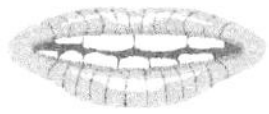

RAPID

F 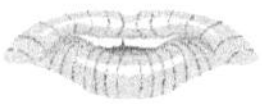

CHANCE

G 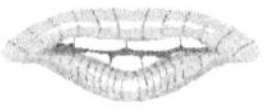

THANK

H 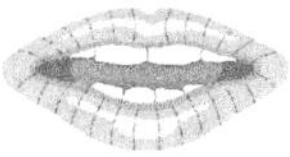

Word puzzle:

	A	*B*	*C*	*D*	*E*	*F*	*G*	*H*	*I*	*J*
1	G	E	R	**R**	A	Y	P	I	D	S
2	R	P	D	A	W	Y	A	**R**	E	N
3	A	M	N	I	L	T	**C**	A	M	E
4	**L**	A	A	**H**	A	R	**G**	A	R	D
5	**T**	R	S	D	**P**	S	S	A	L	**C**
6	**D**	A	Y	N	**G**	**P**	A	N	I	C
7	A	S	T	A	R	H	A	N	C	E
8	**P**	**A**	**C**	**C**	**T**	**C**	R	T	A	**R**
9	E	P	A	R	R	A	E	H	**M**	A
10	L	P	N	A	B	P	T	E	K	R

K.ay.m.	= G3-Came	K.l.ah.s.	= J5-Class
L.ah.j.er.	= A4-Larger	R.ay.l.w.ay.	= D1-Railway
T.ay.s.	= A6-Days	M.ah.k.e.t.	= I9-Market
J.ah.t.s.	= F8-Chance	K.r.a.m.	= D8-Crab
A.m.l.	= B8-Apple	M.ah.s.t.	= A8-Past
K.a.t.t.	= D4-Hand	M.ah.t.ee.	= E5-Party
M.ah.t.	= E8-Trap	R.a.m.i.t.	= H2-Rapid
T.r.a.m.m.	= A5-Tramp	M.a.t.i.k.	= F6-Panic
K.r.a.t.t.	= E6-Grand	K.a.t.	= C8-Can
K.ah.t.e.t.s.	= G4-Gardens	R.ah.th.er.	= J8-Rather

Highlighting:

Instances of lip shape A are underlined/bold:

A very unusual property came onto the m**ar**ket in Cornwall in 2015. It was **a**n old railway c**a**rriage dating from the reign of Queen Victoria **a**nd the early days of the steam railways. When l**a**st used by the Great Western Railway it was a third cl**a**ss c**a**rriage but restored to its original design by a later owner It is now a r**a**ther novel pair of bedrooms **a**nd p**a**rt of l**a**rger bungalow th**a**t h**a**s been built around it **a**nd decorated to look like a Victorian railway station.

Chapter 13 Answers

Nonsense Phrases:

A NEST of strength	=	A test of strength
FEN up to the teeth	=	Fed up to the teeth
WET the chips are down	=	When the chips are down
A DEBT of thieves	=	A den of thieves
DEAD green bottles	=	Ten green bottles
At a TENTER age	=	At a tender age
TENTED pride	=	Dented pride
Pitching a DENT	=	Pitching a tent
Paying the REND	=	Paying the rent
Off to PEN	=	Off to bed
Being LET astray	=	Being led astray

Highlighting lip shape E:

Th**e**re are three species of **e**lephant in the world
They are the **A**sian **e**lephant, the African bush **e**lephant and the African forest **e**lephant
Only the **A**sian **e**lephant has been dom**e**sticated
It can be tr**ai**ned to do m**a**ny kinds of work

The two African species have not been domesticated
The cows live in family groups with their young
They are led by the dominant cow
The bulls, once they have matured, leave the herd
They live alone and meet the cows only for breeding
African **e**lephant numbers are falling due to poaching
Poachers kill the **e**lephants to obt**ai**n their tusks

*Some instances of lip shape E are hidden within the sliding vowels (which we have not yet covered) – full marks if you spotted them in: There, **A**sian, Tr**ai**ned, Their, They, Obt**ai**n*

Chapter 14 Answers

Match the words to the correct lip-shapes

A = Chop B= Stop C=Mop D=Whopper
E=Rubber F=Long G=Frog H=Those

Solution to word puzzle:

	A	B	C	D	E	F	G	H	I	J
1	U	R	Y	R	R	**H**	**O**	O	S	E
2	O	**H**	**S**	**L**	O	O	P	P	P	E
3	N	O	H	O	C	B	E	**O**	**O**	C
4	**L**	O	Y	R	K	A	R	F	F	I
5	**O**	T	T	E	I	T	S	S	**O**	L
6	F	F	**O**	G	N	I	O	O	**J**	I
7	M	E	B	S	D	E	N	R	O	V
8	O	N	U	C	D	N	R	**C**	B	E
9	R	C	R	R	O	F	E	B	B	E
10	**F**	E	E	**T**	**O**	F	**R**	O	Y	R

K.r.o.s.	= H8-Cross	V.r.o.m.	= A10-From
K.o.m.	= F1-Hob	O.t.er.	= B2-Honour
J.o.m.	= I6-Job	L.o.r.ee.	= D2-Lorry
L.o.t.er.ee.	= A4-Lottery	O.m.s.k.ure.	= C6-Obscure
O.v.e.n.s.	= A5-Offence	O.v.er.	= E10-Offer
O.v.i.s.	= H3-Office	O.l.i.v.	= I5-Olive
O.m.oh.s.	= I3-Oppose	R.o.m.er.ee.	= G10-Robbery
J.o.k.i.ng.	= C2-Shocking	T.r.o.t.e.t.	= D10-Trodden
O.m.er.ay.j.u.t.	= G1-Operation		

Chapter 15 Answers

Match the words to the correct lip-shapes

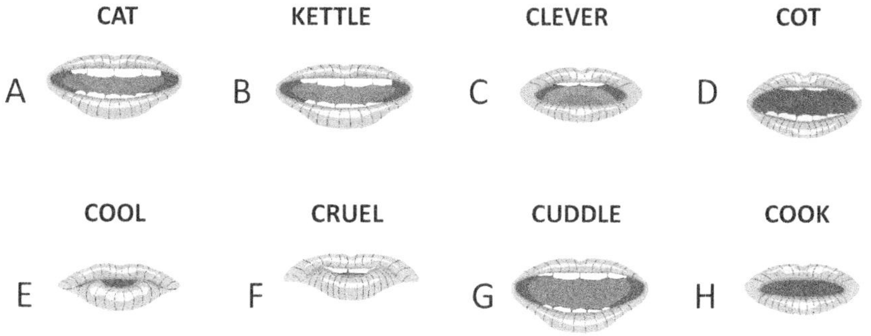
CAT
KETTLE
CLEVER
COT
A
B
C
D
COOL
CRUEL
CUDDLE
COOK
E
F
G
H

Word puzzle:

M.a.k.	= I9-Back	K.ah.m.	= A3-Calm
K.a.r.ee.	= A7-Carry	K.a.j.	= I2-Catch
S.t.i.k.ee.	= D8-Sticky	K.l.e.v.er.	= B10-Clever
K.aw.t.i.t.	= E9-Cornet	K.r.ay.s.ee.	= D2-Crazy
K.r.ee.m.	= A2-Cream	K.r.e.t.i.t.	= I5-Credit
K.ah.t.e.t.	= E4-Garden	K.a.th.er.	= C3-Gather
K.l.ee.m.	= C8-Gleam	K.l.i.t.er.s.	= G4-Glitters
K.r.ay.t.i.t.	= F1-Grated	K.ay.s.t.	= G7-Haste
K.ow.	= B9-How	K.r.i.s.m.us	= J8-Christmas

	A	B	C	D	E	F	G	H	I	J
1	R	E	A	M	Y	**G**	D	R	S	H
2	**C**	L	M	**C**	Z	R	E	E	**C**	C
3	**C**	A	**G**	R	A	A	T	T	A	T
4	H	T	A	N	**G**	A	**G**	T	R	E
5	E	R	Y	E	D	R	L	I	**C**	D
6	A	R	R	**S**	T	I	C	K	T	I
7	**C**	R	L	E	A	M	**H**	Y	C	K
8	V	E	G	E	T	S	A	S	A	**C**
9	E	**H**	O	N	**C**	T	M	A	**B**	H
10	L	**C**	W	R	O	E	T	S	I	R

Chapter 16 Answers

Word puzzle

	A	B	C	D	E	F	G	H	I	J
1	E	S	E	H	H	E	**T**	T	H	E
2	H	L	**C**	T	T	R	H	**O**	**T**	R
3	T	O	**B**	A	A	H	A	T	H	E
4	**R**	A	T	**W**	E	T	**B**	A	T	H
5	O	T	H	E	R	E	O	N	T	H
6	**N**	H	I	N	G	E	**M**	H	A	N
7	**T**	H	O	T	H	**T**	**T**	**T**	K	K
8	**W**	I	R	A	E	M	H	I	C	H
9	H	T	O	E	R	E	**N**	O	R	T
10	H	G	U	**L**	**T**	H	**B**	O	T	H

M.ah.th.	= G4-Bath	M.ay.th.	= C3-Bathe
M.oh.th.	= G10-Both	K.l.oh.th.s.	= C2-Clothes
L.e.th.er.	= D10- Leather	M.u.t.th.	= G6-Month
T.aw.th.	= G9-North	T.u.th.i.ng.	= A6-Nothing
U.th.er.	= H2-Other	R.ah.th.er.	= A4-Rather
T.ee.th.	= F7-Teeth	TH.a.ng.k.	= H7-Thank
TH.a.t.	= G1-That	TH.e.m.	= E10-Them
TH.i.k.	= G7-Thick	TH.u.	= I2-The
TH.u.r.u.	= A7-Thorough	W.e.th.er.	= D4-Weather
W.i.th.	= A8-With		

Lip shapes:

A = Bother B = Thorough C = Fourth D = Weather

Chapter 17 Answers

Nonsense text

There are MANY species of terrapin. SOME live in the warmer PARTS of the United States in fresh or brackish water. They CAN live in SEA water but NEED fresh water TO drink. Fresh water is lighter than salt WATER so in estuaries tends TO stay on the surface. In such circumstances terrapins have BEEN seen to COME to the surface to drink thus avoiding drinking the salty WATER below the surface.

The female terrapin LAYS her eggs in the spring and buries them under the sand. She then goes BACK into the WATER and does NOT return. The eggs incubate and HATCH in the warm sand but the gender of the hatchlings is determined BY the temperature OF the sand IN which they incubate.

People sometimes KEEP terrapins as PETS. In the indoor aquarium their colour is GREEN. In the wild they have a habit of coming out OF the water TO lie in the SUN. This MAKES them much darker in colour.

Word Puzzle:

A.t.i.j.u.t.	= C3-Addition
K.ah.m.e.t.	= A3-Carpet
K.r.ay.t.	= H8-Crane
M.a.ng.k.l.	= F9-Mangle
T.i.t.	= I3-Did
T.o.l.	= B1-Doll
T.r.e.t.	= I7-Dread
V.i.t.l.	= E5-Fiddle
V.u.ng.j.uu.t.	= I5-Function

E.s.t.i.ng.k.t.	= A1-Extinct
K.o.t.t.i.j.t.	= I2-Condition
L.a.t.t.er.n.	= A10-Lantern
M.e.t.ee.	= F1-Penny
T.o.k.	= F3-Knock
T.oh.m.o.t.ee.	= E9-Nobody
T.r.ee.t.	= A6-Treat
V.r.ow.t.	= A7-Frown

	A	B	C	D	E	F	G	H	I	J
1	**E**	**D**	O	K	C	**P**	E	N	D	I
2	X	T	L	L	O	N	N	O	**C**	T
3	**C**	I	**A**	D	D	**K**	N	Y	**D**	I
4	A	N	C	T	I	T	I	D	I	O
5	R	P	E	T	**F**	I	O	N	**F**	N
6	**T**	R	E	A	T	D	A	D	U	N
7	**F**	R	O	E	L	D	E	R	**D**	C
8	N	T	W	N	O	B	O	**C**	N	T
9	A	E	R	N	**N**	**M**	D	R	O	I
10	**L**	E	L	G	N	A	Y	A	N	E

Chapter 18 Answers

Words not ending with lip shape ER:

Car ends with lip shape A (AH)

More ends with lip shape UU (AW)

Matching the words to the correct lip-shapes:

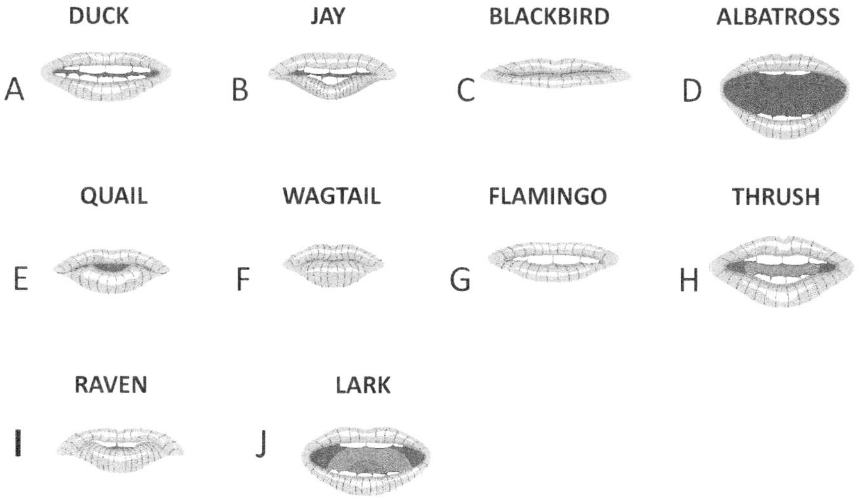
DUCK
JAY
BLACKBIRD
ALBATROSS
A
B
C
D
QUAIL
WAGTAIL
FLAMINGO
THRUSH
E
F
G
H
RAVEN
LARK
I
J

Lip shape text:

M.er.t. = Bird

M.u.r.o.oo = Burrow.

L.o.oo.er. = Lower

K.r.ay.t.l. t.oo. k.r.ay.v. = Cradle to grave

R.a.ee.m. a.n.t. r.ee.s.n. = Rhyme and reason

M.r.a.k.t.l.k.l j.oh.k = Practical joke

Highlighting:

Driving to Mongolia

Three old school friends have set themselves the challenge of driving a Nisan Micra car from London To Mongolia to raise money for charity.

They will be taking part in the Mongol **R**ally over a distance of ten thousand miles.
The money raised will go to the Woking Hospice and also to a charity working to stop rainforest destruction.
The Mongol **R**ally sets out from Battersea Park in July.
The team have mapped out a **r**ough route taking them through Turkey, Georgia, Azerbaijan, Kazakhstan and **R**ussia.
"We are trying not to plan too much as that's part of the fun.
Along the journey they will sleep in the car.

Chapter 19 Answers

Match the words to the correct lip-shapes

SOOT SOUP SEEK

A 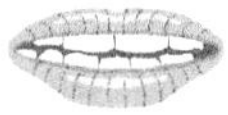 B 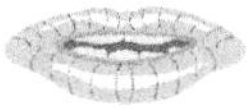 C 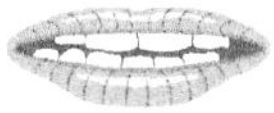

Highlighting:
Voiced S (Z sounds) are in underlined italic type unvoiced S sounds are in **underlined bold**.

STENCILS
Sten**c**il*s* have been around for a very long time
Pre hi**s**toric **s**ten**c**il work ha*s* been found in Argentina
Pre hi**s**toric man'*s* **s**ten**c**il wa*s* hi*s* hand
He **s**pat ink through it onto the cave wall
Sten**c**il*s* can be made from mo**s**t thin material*s*
If they are **s**trong enough they can be u*s*ed many time*s*
It i*s* not po**ss**ible to make every shape u*s*ing a **s**imple **s**ten**c**il
A **s**ten**c**il to print the shape of the letter O will fall apart

Thi**s** is because the **c**entral part is an island
It is not connected to the re**s**t of the **s**ten**c**il
To overcome thi**s** problem **s**ten**c**ils are made with bridges
These connect the islands to the re**s**t of the **s**ten**c**il
The bridges also prevent the ink from getting to the paper
They leave gap**s** in the printed letters

The printed S of island is not a spoken S.

The printed S in 'shape' is a different lip shape.

Word puzzle:

	A	B	C	D	E	F	G	H	I	J
1	P	P	E	R	X	I	U	**S**	C	I
2	U	L	**S**	I	A	M	N	S	K	R
3	**S**	A	N	G	**M**	U	A	C	K	**T**
4	P	U	O	C	K	M	**S**	D	E	N
5	**S**	O	**S**	W	I	**S**	U	D	E	**T**
6	E	L	**S**	**T**	C	E	**N**	I	C	A
7	**S**	G	L	**P**	E	A	C	E	I	X
8	I	N	I	E	N	C	E	**S**	E	A
9	E	P	P	I	E	S	S	O	N	L
10	R	Y	**S**	C	R	**P**	**S**	O	D	E

M.a.s.i.m.u.m. = E3-Maximum

M.ee.s. = D7-Peace

M.r.e.s. = F10-Press

T.w.ii.s.	= D6-Twice	S.a.k.	= G4-Sack
S.ee.l.t.	= H8-Sealed	S.i.k.t.uu.l.	= C2-Signal
S.i.ng.k.l.	= A7-Single	S.ii.u.t.s.	= C10-Science
S.l.i.m.er.ee.	= C6-Slippery	S.o.k.	= C5-Sock
S.oo.m.	= A5-Soup	S.oo.t.	= G10-Soon
S.u.m.er.	= A3-Supper	S.u.t.	= H1-Sun
S.u.t.t.	= F5-Sudden	T.a.s.ee.	= J5-Taxi
T.ii.s.	= G6-Nice	T.r.i.k.s.	= J3-Tricks

Chapter 20 Answers:

Lookalikes:

Shop/Chop	Jane/Shane/Chain
Fletch/Fledge/Flesh	Jib/Ship/Chip
Jaw/Chore/Shore	Mash/Badge/Match
Catch/Cash/Cadge	Jean/Cheat/Sheet/Sheen.

Highlighting: *(Those in italic vary from person to person.)*

Deep fried fi**sh** was intro***duc***ed to England in the sixteenth century
It was sold by Jewi**sh** refu**g**ees from the continent
Fi**sh** and **ch**ips was a popular working class di**sh** in the nineteenth cen*t*ury
This was because trawl fi**sh**ing produced a plentiful supply of fre**sh** fi**sh**
Deep fried **ch**ips first appeared in England in eighteen sixty
They were sold in London by Joseph Malin a Jewi**sh** refu**g**ee
During World War Two fi**sh** and **ch**ips was exempt from ra**tio**ning
but **ch**ip **sh**op customers had to bring their own newspaper
Tradi**tio**nal frying uses beef dripping or lard

however, ve**g**etable oils, are often used instead
American style Fren**ch** fries are thinner than Engli**sh** **ch**ips
The lar**g**er surface area absorbs more fat.

Chapter 21 Answers

Nonsense text:

Yorkshire Pudding was described in eighteenth century cook books as **dripping** pudding.
It was served as the **first** course of a **meal** to dampen the appetite.
This was so that **diners** would require less **meat** in the following **course**.
It was a **money** saving practice **in** households that were **not** so well **off**.
In even poorer households there was **no** meat course and Yorkshire Pudding was the **meal**.
It was a **means** of producing a nourishing **meal** using only dripping, **flour,** milk and eggs.
It is believed **that** its association with the county of Yorkshire was because **of** the availability of **cheap** coal.
Burning **coal** produced the high temperatures required **for** making Yorkshire Pudding **which** was often served with gravy.

Lip shape text:

K.e.l.m. y.aw.s.e.l.v.	= Help yourself
W.o.t. u. k.a.r.ee. o.t.	= What a carry-on
Y.u.ng. a.t.t. m.ew.t.i.v.uu.l.	= Young and beautiful
U. l.u.v.l.ee. k.o.l.i.t.ay.	= A lovely holiday
EW.j.ew.u.l. m.r.ii.s.	= Usual price
V.ah.s.t. a.t.t. v.ure.ee.u.s.	= Fast and furious

Y.aw.k.j.u. m.uu.t.i.ng. = Yorkshire pudding

S.t.o.m. w.u.r.ee.i.ng. = Stop worrying

Word puzzle:

	A	B	C	D	E	F	G	H	I	J
1	A	R	L	Y	E	M	I	**F**	U	R
2	**E**	**Y**	E	A	S	T	T	R	A	Y
3	D	A	Y	O	**D**	A	Y	**U**	E	**Y**
4	I	U	R	I	**S**	**C**	A	S	U	A
5	L	**C**	S	E	E	C	R	**Y**	A	L
6	O	**H**	**U**	T	S	U	R	**Y**	R	D
7	D	A	**L**	H	E	R	Y	O	U	T
8	Y	**E**	A	C	A	**Y**	G	U	F	H
9	B	D	S	L	Y	**L**	N	L	**W**	O
10	I	R	Y	E	V	O	I	Y	R	R

K.a.r.ee. = F4-Carry

T.ay.t.ii.m.= E3-Daytime

EE.s.ee. = B8-Easy

L.u.v.l.ee. = F9-Lovely

EW.s. = C6-Use

Y.ah.t. = H5-Yard

Y.ee.s.t. = B2-Yeast

K.ure.ee.oh. = B5-Curio

ER.l.ee. = A2-Early

V.ure.ee. = H1-Fury

S.e.k.ure. = E4-Secure

EW.j.ew.u.l. = H3-Usual

Y.er. = J3-Year

Y.o.t.s. = F8-Yachts

K.o.l.i.t.ay. = B6-Holiday

L.ay.t.ee.m.er.t. = C7-Ladybird

W.u.r.ee.i.ng. = I9-Worrying

Y.oo.th.v.uu.l. = H6-Youthful

Chapter 22 Answers

Word Puzzle:

	A	B	C	D	E	F	G	H
1	E	V	Y	H	O	W	**F**	R
2	N	**A**	R	**S**	H	O	U	I
3	U	E	**T**	**C**	**S**	U	R	A
4	E	**C**	H	R	O	T	Y	**P**
5	C	I	O	**C**	W	D	**C**	L
6	E	**N**	A	R	N	R	A	E
7	W	**E**	N	**A**	I	A	R	**B**
8	**C**	U	E	I	D	**C**	A	R
9	H	R	O	P	**C**	E	R	E
10	A	I	N	E	H	E	R	E

A.v.e.n.ew.= B2-Avenue
B.r.ay.n. = H7-Brain
C.r.ay.n. = D5-Crane
CH.ia. = E9-Cheer
F.ure.ee. = G1-Fury
K.r.ow.d. = D3-Crowd
N.ew. = B6-New
SH.ow.t. = E3-Shout
URE.oh.p. = B7-Europe

AY.d. = D7-Aid
C.l.ia. = G5-Clear
CH.ay.n. = A8-Chain
CH.oi.s. = B4-Choice
K.a.r.ia. = F8-Career
M.air = H4-Pair
SH.oh.w. = D2-Show
T.r.ii. = C3-Try

Match the words to the correct lip-shape sequences:

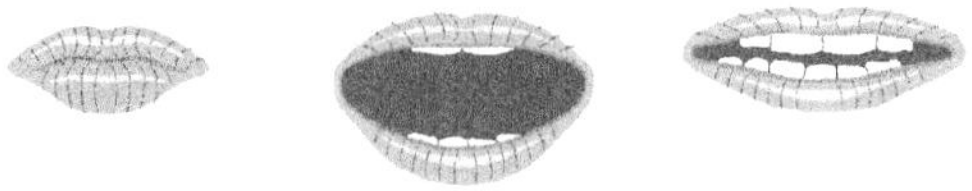

= Why

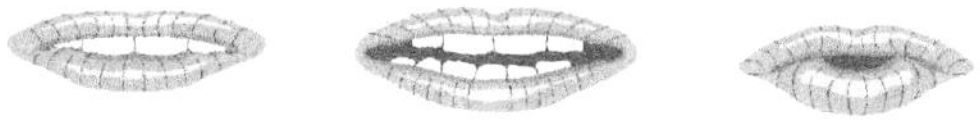

= Few

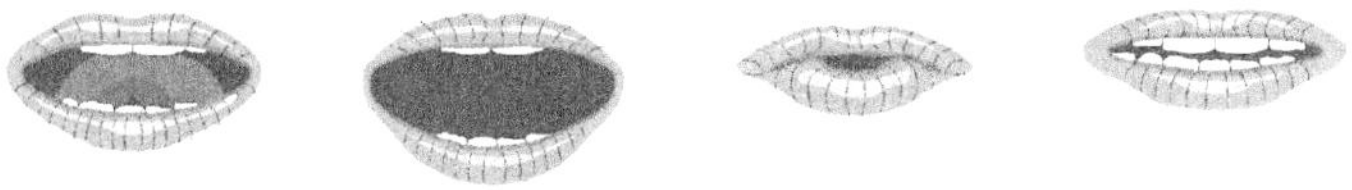

= Loud

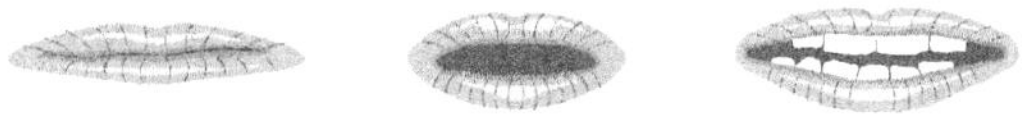

= Boy

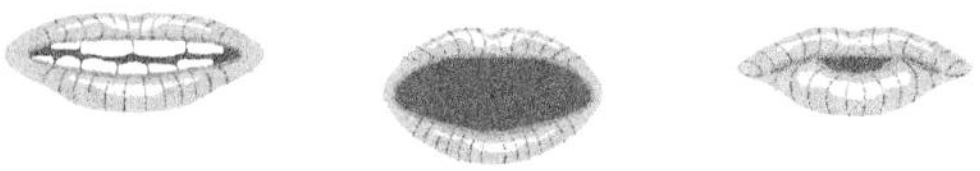

= Know

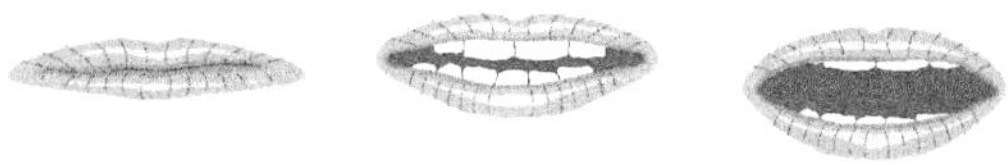

= Pier

Chapter 23 Answers

The lip shapes are saying the word: Shoot

Match the words to the correct lip-shapes

OVER OUNCE EWE VIEW

A 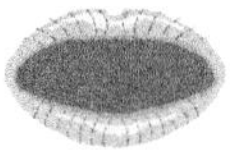 B 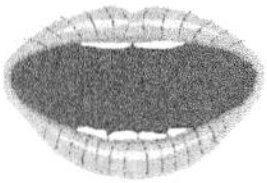 C 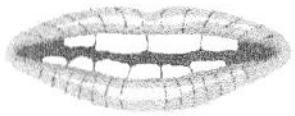 D 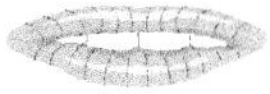

Highlighting

D day anniversary
Bernard Jordan, was a ninety year **ol**d veteran of world war t**wo**.
He made the headlines last J**u**ne when he went missing from his nursing h**o**me.
He was discovered later in France at the D day celebrations.
Sadly, Bernard died back in Jan**u**ary.
His medals came up at auction some time later.
They fetched one th**ou**sand seven hundred and fifty p**ou**nds.
The British buyer of the medals lives in Normandy.
He intends to put them on public display in the shop he runs.

Word Puzzle

J.ow.t.	= E10-Shout	K.er.v.ew.	= A1-Curfew
K.r.ow.l.	= E9-Growl	K.r.ow.t.	= E4-Crowd
K.r.oo.t	= A10-Crude	K.r.oo.v.	= B6-Groove
M.l.oh.t.	= B1-Bloat	M.l.oo.	= F5-Blue
M.oh.t.	= G9-Moat	M.r.ow.t.	= B1-Brown
R.ow.t.t.	= G5-Round	T.ow.er.	= D6-Tower
T.ew.	= E3-Dew	T.r.ow.t.	= G4-Trout
T.r.oo.m.	= A7-Troop	V.ew.	= D2-Few
V.oh.k.	= G7-Folk		

	A	B	C	D	E	F	G	H
1	**C**	**B**	A	O	L	**B**	U	T
2	U	R	T	**F**	E	W	O	D
3	R	O	W	N	**D**	E	R	N
4	F	W	O	R	**C**	W	**T**	U
5	E	D	E	U	L	**B**	**R**	O
6	W	**G**	R	**T**	O	W	E	R
7	**T**	R	O	O	V	E	**F**	T
8	E	O	O	P	K	L	O	A
9	D	U	U	T	**G**	R	**M**	O
10	**C**	R	O	H	**S**	O	W	L

Chapter 24 Answers

Match the words to the correct lip-shapes

LEARN
A 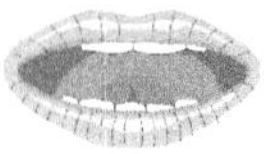

PAIR
B 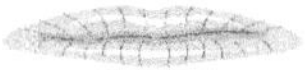

GEAR
C 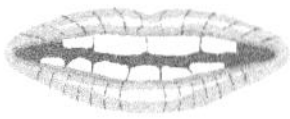

FAIR
D 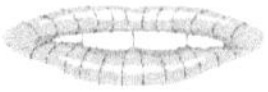

CARE
E 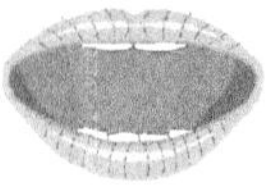

WEIR
F 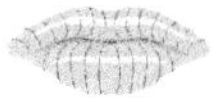

URCHIN
G 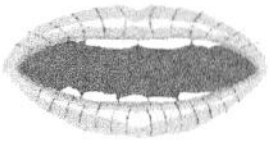

JOURNEY
H 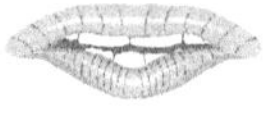

Word puzzle:

A.m.j.air. = H3-Armchair

ER.l.ee. = C10-Early

K.air. = I4-Care

M.ay.m.er. = J1-Paper

R.e.m.air. = A7-Repair

S.er.v.i.s. = A4-Service

S.t.er.t. = E3-Stern

U.m.s.t.air.s.=B1-Upstairs

A.w.air. = H7-Aware

J.air. = G3-Share

K.er.l.ee. = A3-Curly

M.er.v.ew.m.= E4-Perfume

R.e.t.er.t.s. = B10-Returns

S.er.v.t. = B5-Served

TH.r.e.t.m.air.
= F7-Threadbare

V.er.th.er. = H8-Further

	A	B	C	D	E	F	G	H	I	J
1	S	**U**	P	S	N	R	E	P	A	**P**
2	R	I	A	T	R	E	H	A	R	E
3	**C**	U	R	L	**S**	T	**S**	**A**	R	M
4	**S**	E	R	Y	**P**	R	I	A	H	C
5	E	**S**	V	I	E	E	R	A	**C**	A
6	R	V	E	C	R	F	U	W	E	R
7	**R**	E	D	E	H	**T**	M	**A**	R	T
8	A	P	U	R	R	E	E	**F**	U	H
9	I	E	T	N	S	A	D	B	E	E
10	R	**R**	**E**	A	R	L	Y	A	R	R

Chapter 25 Answers

Nonsense Text:

Oranges are a delicious fruit containing **an** abundance of vitamin **C**. **Once** the juicy inner **part** has been eaten **it** is usual **to** simply discard the outer **peel**. But the **peel** of your orange has **some** uses you **might** not have thought **of.** It has a pleasant citrus fragrance which **has** led to **its** use as an air freshener. You simply leave **it** lying around in some inconspicuous **place**. Some people have used **it** as a body scrub when taking a shower. Other have rubbed **it** on their **skin** to deter mosquitoes. Orange skin is edible and **can** be used candied as cake fruit **or** as a delicious **snack**. **It** can be infused in **hot** water to make orange **tea**. The aromatic oils **it** contains will infuse into olive oil if left **to** soak for a few days- the oil **can** then be used **as** a salad dressing.

Word Puzzle:

	A	B	C	D	E	F	G	H
1	I	**O**	**A**	L	**J**	O	I	N
2	L	Y	P	U	N	**A**	M	E
3	**W**	L	P	F	N	**T**	I	R
4	E	I	O	Y	O	Y	E	E
5	**R**	R	**J**	U	C	S	R	A
6	E	W	D	E	**S**	E	**R**	**C**
7	N	E	G	H	H	A	M	E
8	**W**	E	I	**S**	T	**B**	E	T
9	E	D	**S**	E	E	E	R	R
10	L	I	O	D	I	**H**	Y	A

J.ay.m.	= E6-Shame	J.oi.t.	= E1-Join
J.oi.v.uu.l.	= C5-Joyful	K.ii.t.	= F10-Hide
K.a.r.ear.	= H6-Career	M.i.t.r.ay.	= F8-Betray
R.e.s.k.ew.t.	= G5-Rescued	R.e.t.ew.	= A5-Renew
S.t.ear.	= D8-Steer	S.oi.l.t.	= C9-Soiled
T.ii.m.	= F3-Time	U.m.l.ii.	= C`-Apply
U.t.oi.	= F2-Annoy	Ol.l.	= B1-Oil
W.ay.	= A8-Weigh	W.ear.= A3-Weir	

Highlighting: Fresh-water Eels

There are **nineteen** **species** of fresh-water **eels** in the world.
They have long **snake-like** bodies but although **they** look **like** **snakes** **they** are in fact fish.
The **European** fresh-water **eel** spends part of its **life** in the **sea**
An **eel** also spends part of its **life** in fresh-water **streams**, rivers and **lakes.**
Its **life** begins in the Sargasso **Sea** where as a **juvenile** its **body** is small and transparent
When it has grown large enough to **be** recognised as an **eel** but is still transparent it called a glass **eel**
Glass **eels** **migrate** to river estuaries where **they** experience a **mixture** of salt water and fresh-water on a regular **cycle**.
During this **time** they stop **being** transparent and **take** on the colour of and adult **eel**
Once **they** have colour **they** are known as elvers and **migrate** **upstream**.
They spend the **main** part of their **lives** in fresh-water.
The **final** episode in the **life** of an **eel** is to return to the Sargasso **Sea** to spawn and give **rise** to the next generation of fresh-water **eels**.

Chapter 26 Answers

Highlight instances of lip shape II:

The use of ink for writing began about four thousand five hundred years ago.

The first kind of ink invented was made from lamp black mixed with vegetable oil.

The carbon rich lamp black gave a strong colour that would not fade in the light..

The oil enabled the ink to flow and as it soaked into the writing surface left a sticky deposit enabling the lamp black to adhere.

Indian ink was invented by the Chinese in the fourth century before Christ.

It was made by combining lamp black with ground up charred bones mixed with animal glue.

This was a water based type of ink that could be stored as a solid and mixed with water when it was needed for writing.

It formed a strong bond with the writing surface that does not fade over time.

Match the words to the correct lip-shapes:

EAT IMP EYE EARN

A B C D

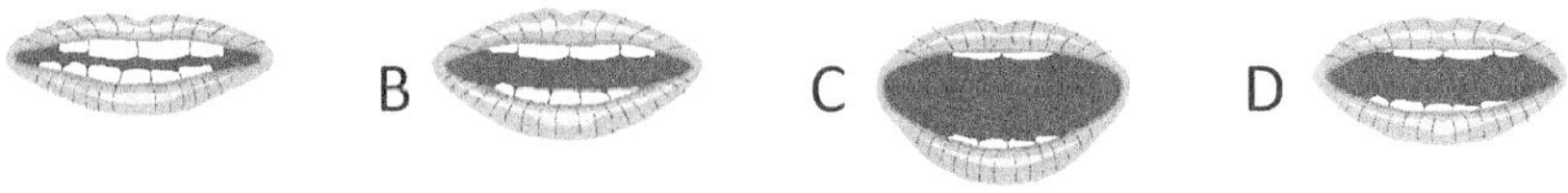

Chapter 27 Answers

Match the words to the correct lip-shapes:

The lip-shape pictures show the first lip-shape seen when the following words are spoken:

FOOTBALL	RUGBY	GOLF	SHINTY
A 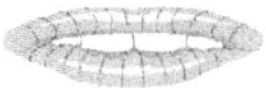	B 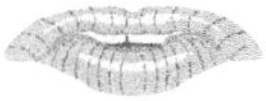	C 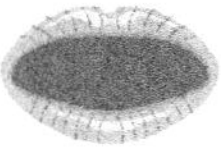	D 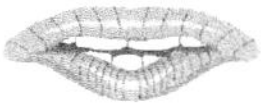

LAWN BOWLS	WATER POLO	STICKBALL	HOOVERBALL
E 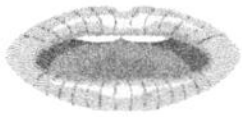	F 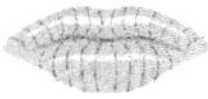	G 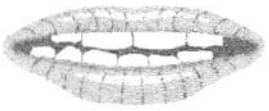	H 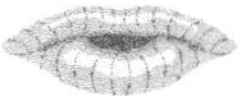

Answers to word puzzle:

F.i.ng.g.er. = A3-Finger
A.ng.k.l. = I1-Ankle
L.a.ng.g.w.i.j. = B2-Language
B.r.i.ng.k. = Brink
B.l.a.ng.k. = C2-Blank
M.i.ng.g.l. = C6-Mingle
F.u.ng.g.u.s. = C7-Fungus
B.l.a.ng.k.i.t. = J3-Blanket
D.o.ng.k.ee. = D3-Donkey
TH.i.ng.k. = D9-Think
A.ng.g.r.ee. = D5-Angry
H.u.ng.g.r.ee. = B7-Hungry
P.e.n.n.ii.f. = D7-Penknife
CH.i.ng.k. = H4-Chink
E.l.o.ng.g.ay.t. = H1-Elongate

	A	B	C	D	E	F	G	H	I	J
1	N	G	E	R	N	K	Y	**E**	**A**	N
2	I	**L**	**B**	L	A	K	E	L	L	K
3	**F**	A	E	**D**	O	N	N	O	E	**B**
4	G	N	L	E	T	A	G	**C**	H	L
5	U	N	G	**A**	N	G	K	N	I	A
6	A	I	**M**	E	N	R	Y	E	T	N
7	G	**H**	**F**	**P**	K	N	I	F	E	K
8	E	U	U	H	I	**B**	R	I	G	L
9	G	N	N	**T**	N	K	K	N	N	E
10	R	Y	G	U	S	**E**	N	T	A	D

Chapter 28 Answers

Lip shape pictures:

A = Leisure
B = Fury
C = Mature

Word puzzle:

A.t.v.e.t.j.ure.	=	E8-Adventure
V.ay.l.ure.	=	A1-Failure
A.m.a.t.ure.	=	C1-Amateur
V.ee.oo.t.ure.	=	D2-Future
A.j.ure.u.t.s.	=	H8-Assurance
T.ay.t.ure.	=	J5-Nature
S.e.t.t.ure.ee.u.t.	=	E5-Centurion

O.m.s.k.ure. = A9-Obscure
O.m.s.k.ure.i.t.ee. = C6-Obscurity
S.e.t.t.ure.ee. = H1-Century
K.r.ee.t.ure. = B1-Creature
M.i.k.t.ure. = A8-Picture
K.ure.ee.o.s.i.t.ee. = D1-Curiosity

	A	B	C	D	E	F	G	H	I	J
1	**F**	**C**	R	**C**	U	R	**A**	**C**	E	N
2	A	E	E	**F**	E	I	M	A	Y	T
3	I	R	A	U	R	O	E	T	R	U
4	L	U	T	T	U	S	R	E	U	R
5	E	R	U	Y	**C**	I	U	T	A	**N**
6	S	B	**O**	T	E	T	Y	I	O	N
7	C	U	R	I	N	T	U	R	N	C
8	**P**	I	E	R	**A**	D	S	**A**	A	E
9	**O**	C	T	U	E	V	S	U	R	E
10	B	S	C	U	R	E	N	T	U	R

Chapter 29 Answers

The lip shapes say:

A=Above B=Appeal C= Really D=Junior

Highlighting:

Mary is fourteen years old.

She was born deaf and has no cochl<u>**ea**</u> in either ear and no auditory nerve either.

Th<u>e</u> cochl<u>ea</u> is <u>a</u> small, snail shaped part of the inner ear

that turns sound waves into nerve signals.
These are normally sent on to the brain through the auditory nerve, but Mary has no auditory nerve.
To correct his problem Mary received an auditory brainstem implant.
The implant turns sound into electrical signals which are fed directly into her brain.
Mary can now hear and take part in normal conversation even though she has no cochleas or auditory nerves
Many deaf people are able to hear again after a cochlear implant operation.
Mary is the first to have an implant that links directly to the brain stem.

Word puzzle solution:

	A	B	C	D	E	F	G	H	I	J
1	**D**	**C**	**P**	A	T	I	**P**	**D**	E	L
2	O	R	E	C	N	E	R	U	S	I
3	V	U	M	B	L	C	E	O	I	C
4	E	**B**	U	S	E	I	N	T	A	L
5	U	S	T	A	R	O	E	**R**	S	H
6	**C**	**C**	U	**C**	D	U	**D**	U	I	D
7	Y	R	R	U	P	S	**L**	B	B	N
8	D	E	R	**S**	**L**	O	O	N	D	U
9	N	T	A	T	**U**	V	E	N	O	O
10	**U**	I	O	N	N	D	E	R	G	R

K.r.u.m.m.l.- = B1-Crumble
K.u.r.ee. = B6-Curry
T.e.l.i.j.u.s.- = H1-Delicious
T.u.v. - = A1-Dove
L.u.v. = E8-Love
M.ay.j.u.t.s. = C1-Patience
R.u.m.i.j. = H5-Rubbish
U.n.t.er. = A10-Under
U.n.t.er.k.r.ow.n.t. = E9-Underground

K.u.m.- = D6-Cup
K.u.s.t.ah.t. = A1-Custard
T.e.n.t.u.l. = G6-Dental
L.u.n.t.u.n.- = G7-London
M.u.s.- = B4-Bus
M.r.e.j.u.s.- = G1-Precious
S.t.ay.j.u.n. = D8-Station

Chapter 30

Answers -

Word puzzle:

	A	B	C	D	E	F	G	H
1	F	L	E	L	D	O	I	C
2	**Y**	O	S	U	**C**	H	**A**	E
3	L	U	R	O	H	**S**	N	N
4	A	U	D	D	**S**	P	O	O
5	Y	**P**	**C**	I	N	G	I	Y
6	O	**R**	L	**G**	W	E	L	**C**
7	**B**	**C**	A	N	A	R	O	H
8	U	O	W	**M**	O	**L**	O	Y
9	T	U	L	D	R	A	**B**	L
10	C	H	E	R	E	W	F	U

M.uu.j.er. = A7-Butcher
K.uu.t. = B7-Could
M.uu.t.i.ng. = B5-Pudding
U.n.uu.ee. = G2-Annoy
J.uu.ee.s. = E2-Choice
L.uu.v.uu.l. = F8-Lawful
J.uu.t. = E4-Should
Y.uu.s.e.l.v. = A2-Yourself

K.l.uu. = C5-Claw
M.uu. = D8-More
R.uu.ee.y.a.l.= B6-Royal
M.uu.ee. = G9-Boy
N.uu. = D6-Gnaw
J.uu. = H6-Chore
S.m.uu.ee.l. = F3-Spoil

Highlighting lip shape UU:

Put your foot in it
Little **choice**
More choice
Foot in the **door**
Food **for thought**
Claw back
Good look

Could you come
Choice of words
Oily rag
Good morning
Short fuse
Good book
Calling card

Lip shape sequences:

A = Yourself   B = Awful   C = Boil
D = Boy   E = Spoil   F = Pudding

Chapter 31 Answers

Quiz on the McGurk Effect:

Which statements about the McGurk effect are true – select one or more:

A. The McGurk effect works only with hard-of-hearing people.
__Incorrect__ – the effect works with most people irrespective of whether they have a hearing deficiency.

B. The McGurk effect does not work with vowel sounds.
__Incorrect__ – the effect works with vowels but not so well as with consonant sounds.

C. Works if speaker and listener use different languages.
Correct

D. Stops working if sound and vision do not match.
__Incorrect__ -the effect works because sound and vision do not match.

F. Works with teenagers.
__Correct__ – it also works with other age groups.

G. Can be switched on and off at will.
   Incorrect – *The effect is involuntary, it takes place in the subconscious mind.*

Chapter 32 Answers

Which of these statements is correct? Select one or more.

A. High sounds travel faster than low sounds. ***Incorrect***
B. Low sounds are better at going round corners than high sounds. ***Correct***
C. Quiet sounds travel slower than loud sounds. ***Incorrect***
D. Sounds from the left are quieter in the right ear and louder in the left ear. ***Correct***
E. Sounds from the left reach the right ear a fraction later than the left ear receives them. ***Correct***
F. A person who is totally deaf in one ear cannot discern the direction sounds come from. ***Correct***
G. Head shadow is the area sounds cannot reach. ***Incorrect***

Chapter 33 Answers

Fill in the blanks to complete the sentences.

The ability for people to follow one particular voice against background noise is called the **Cocktail party effect**.

If you can see the lips of the speaker but not see the source of the background noise the **Ventriloquism effect** will help you to distinguish the voice of the speaker from the background noise.

A1. Table of phonetic symbols:

Phonetic symbols are in bold type.

A as in hat	**N** as in nail
AH as in car	**NG** as in Thing
AIR as in care	**O** as in Hot
AW as in claw	**OH** as in Crow
AY as in hay	**OI** as in Boy
B as in box	**OO** as in Cool
C as in cat	**OW** as in Cow
CH as in choice	**P** as in Post
D as in dog	**Q** as in Queen
E as in tent	**R** as in Rat
EAR as in clear	**S** as in Silver
EE as in feet	**SH** as in Ship
ER as in hurt	**T** as in Tiger
EW as in few	**TH** as in thick
F as in Fig	**U** as in cup
G as in goat	**URE** as in pure
H as in hot	**UU** as in foot
I as in lip	**V** as in vast
IA as in idea	**W** as in wax
II as in cry	**X** as in box
J as in jam	**Y** as in year
L as in list	**Z** as in zoo
M as in make	**ZH** as in decision

A2. Primary lip shapes:

Lip Shape **A (hat)** for A,AH and OW1 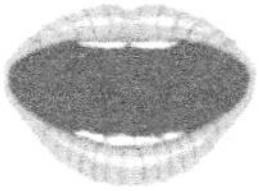	Lip Shape **E (tent)** for E,AY1 and AIR1 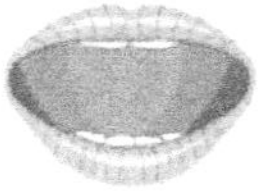	Lip Shape **EE (feet)** for EE, AY2, EW1 IA1, II2 and OI2 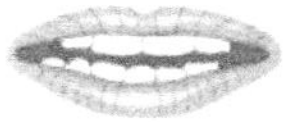	Lip Shape **ER (hurt)** for ER and AiR2 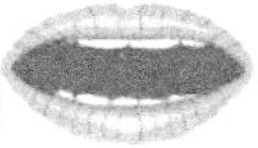
Lip Shape **I (lip)** for I 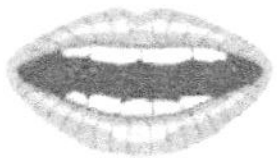	Lip Shape J for CH, J, SH and ZH 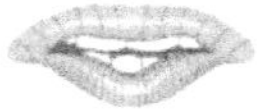	Lip Shape **K** for C, G, H and K 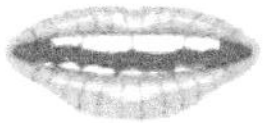	Lip Shape **L** for L 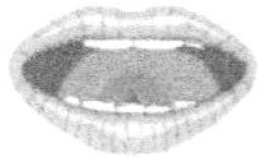
Lip Shape **M** for B, M and P 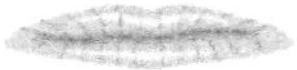	Lip Shape **O (hot)** for O and OH1 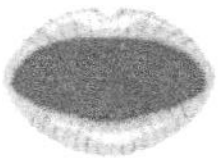	Lip Shape **OO (too)** for OO, EW2, OH2 and OW2 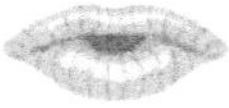	Lip Shape **R** for R and URE3 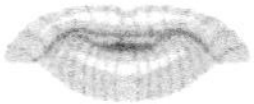
Lip Shape **S** for S,X and Z 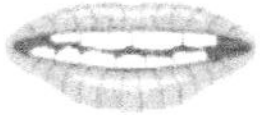	Lip Shape **T** for T, D and N 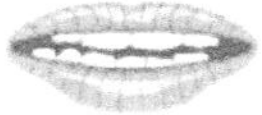	Lip Shape **TH** For TH 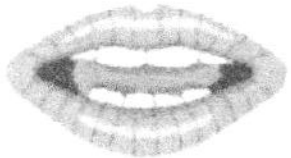	Lip Shape **U (cup)** for U and IA2 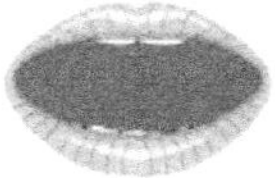
Lip Shape **UU (put)** for AW, OI1, URE2 and UU 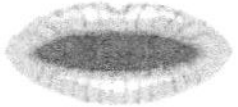	Lip Shape **V** for F and V 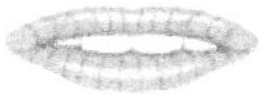	Lip Shape **W** for Q and W 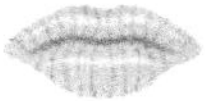	Lip Shape **Y** for Y and URE1 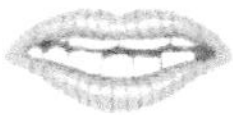

A3. Sliding lip shapes:

- the lips change from the first shape to the next shape while the sound is being made

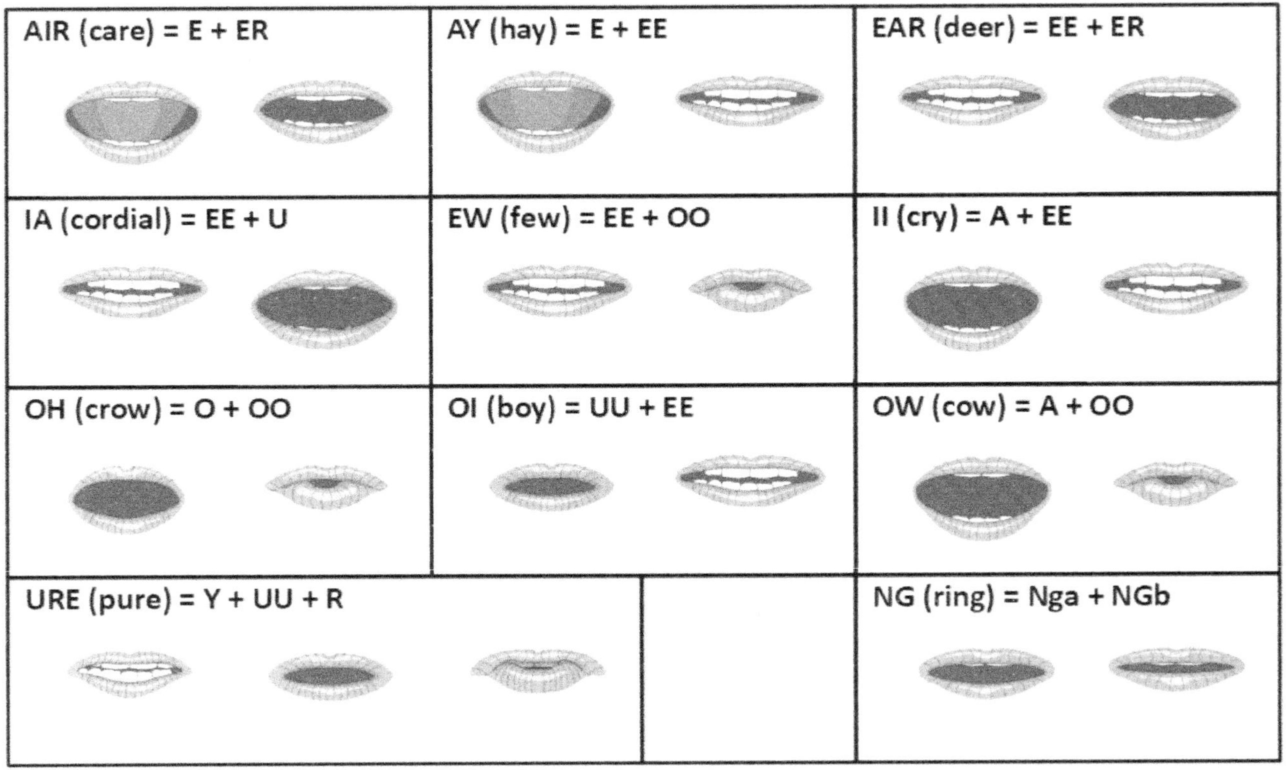
AIR (care) = E + ER
AY (hay) = E + EE
EAR (deer) = EE + ER
IA (cordial) = EE + U
EW (few) = EE + OO
II (cry) = A + EE
OH (crow) = O + OO
OI (boy) = UU + EE
OW (cow) = A + OO
URE (pure) = Y + UU + R
NG (ring) = Nga + NGb

A4. Phonetic text to lip shape conversion table:

Phonetic Symbol	Lip Shape(s)	Phonetic Symbol	Lip Shape(s)
A	A	**N**	T
AH	A	**NG**	NG
AIR	E.ER	**O**	O
AW	UU	**OH**	O.OO
AY	E.EE	**OI**	UU.EE
B	M	**OO**	OO
C	K	**OW**	A.OO
CH	J	**P**	M
D	T	**Q**	W
E	E	**R**	R
EAR	EE.ER	**S**	S
EE	EE	**SH**	J
ER	ER	**T**	T
EW	EE.OO	**TH**	TH
F	V	**U**	U
G	K	**URE**	Y.UU.R
H	K	**UU**	UU
I	I	**V**	V
IA	EE.U	**W**	W
II	A.EE	**X**	S
J	J	**Y**	Y
K	K	**Z**	S
L	L	**ZH**	J
M	M		

A5. Basic Lip Shape Text *- reference table*

Lip shape	Sound(s)	Lip shape	Sound(s)
A	A, AH	**O**	O
AIR	AIR	**OH**	OH
AY	AY	**OI**	OI
E	E	**OO**	OO
EAR	EAR	**OW**	OW
EE	EE	**R**	R
ER	ER	**S**	S, X, Z
EW	EW	**T**	T, D, N
I	I	**TH**	TH
IA	IA	**U**	U
II	II	**URE**	URE
J	J, CH, SH, ZH	**UU**	UU, AW
K	K, C, G, H	**V**	V, F
L	L	**W**	W, Q
M	M, P, B	**Y**	Y
NG	NG		

A6. Advanced Lip Shape Text

Lip shape(s) to sound(s) conversion table

Lip Shape(s)	Sound(s)	Lip Shape(s)	Sound(s)
A	A, AH	**O**	O
E.ER	AIR	**O.OO**	OH
E.EE	AY	**UU.EE**	OI
E	E	**OO**	OO
EE.ER	EAR	**A.OO**	OW
EE	EE	**R**	R
ER	ER	**S**	S, X, Z
EE.OO	EW	**T**	T, D, N
I	I	**TH**	TH
EE.U	IA	**U**	U
A.EE	II	**Y.UU.R**	URE
J	J, CH, SH, ZH	**UU**	UU, AW
K	K, C, G, H	**V**	V, F
L	L	**W**	W, Q
M	M, P, B	**Y**	Y
NGa.NGb	NG		